50 THINGS YOU SHOULD KNOW ABOUT THE CHRONIC FATIGUE SYNDROME EPIDEMIC

Printed in the United States of America.
First Edition

Cover photograph by Robert Bruce Eves.

Library of Congress Cataloguing-in-Publication Data

Ostrom, Neenyah
  50 Things You Should Know About The Chronic Fatigue Syndrome Epidemic
  I. Title

Library of Congress Catalog Card Number: 91-068145

ISBN: 0-9624142-2-0

TNM, Inc.
P.O. Box 1475
Church Street Station
New York, NY 10008

50 THINGS YOU SHOULD KNOW ABOUT THE CHRONIC FATIGUE SYNDROME EPIDEMIC

Contents

Chronic Fatigue Syndrome is, right now, almost impossible to diagnose when it first begins, because it often appears to be identical to the flu.

One of the biggest drawbacks to the name "Chronic Fatigue Syndrome" is that the syndrome—a collection of many symptoms—can become confused with a single symptom: being chronically fatigued.

With CFS, the patient's immune system doesn't work the way it should—it is dysfunctional.

All too often, when a patient with undiagnosed CFS goes to a doctor to find out what is wrong, the patient will be told that he or she has depression.

Research is increasingly showing that CFS is a contagious illness; that is, an illness which can be spread from one person to another, in an as-yet-unknown manner.

For a number of years, people with CFS have suspected that their pets—dogs, cats, even horses—were coming down with CFS, too.

Dr. David Bell has studied an outbreak of epidemic CFS—which included a number of children—in Lyndonville, New York.

Anyone can catch CFS, "including children," according to Ottawa physician Dr. Byron Hyde, "after contact with a person coughing in the elevator or in the next aircraft seat."

Introduction

America is facing a health crisis of unprecedented proportions, a crisis that has been misleadingly labeled Chronic Fatigue Syndrome. This health crisis has been bungled by government health officials from the very beginning: It has been ignored, misrepresented, and investigated ineptly until, as I write this in January 1992, untold millions of Americans already have contracted this potentially disabling, AIDS-like illness.

I have written about Chronic Fatigue Syndrome, or CFS, since February 1988—before the illness was officially recognized by U.S. health agencies. Over the years, investigating the epidemic for a newspaper called the *New York Native*, I have talked with countless victims of CFS and have witnessed, first-hand, the tragedies that have befallen them as a result of this illness.

I have watched relationships dissolve, careers crumble, and CFS patients brought to the brink of homelessness because they suffer from an illness that the U.S. government refuses to investigate seriously. As a result, public and private disability insurers also refuse to admit that CFS is a debilitating illness, and desperately ill CFS patients are left with no place to turn for help.

I have also witnessed the bungling of the investigation of this epidemic by the people entrusted with protecting the public health of the nation: the Centers for Disease Control and the National Institutes of Health. It took the Centers for Disease Control almost four years to recognize CFS as a "real" disease. And the most important CFS researcher at the National Institutes of Health continues to assert that CFS is a form of depression—in the face of evidence that it is an illness of profound immune system dysfunction that shares a disturbing number of characteristics with AIDS.

The activist movement that has arisen during the AIDS epidemic has demonstrated that private individuals can affect public health policy. A similar activist movement has arisen all over the country as CFS patients have realized that they cannot depend on the medical establishment or U.S. health agencies to protect

13

or assist them.

CFS is clearly an AIDS-related illness that puts the entire world population at risk. In contrast to the disdain with which CFS has been treated by U.S. health authorities, scientists in other countries—Britain, Canada, New Zealand, Australia, Germany, and Japan—have investigated CFS with utmost seriousness.

This book is a call to action to the citizens of the United States to speak out against the inaction of the U.S. government in the face of an epidemic that has already destroyed the lives and livelihoods of millions of Americans.

The efforts of some government health officials to suppress information about the severity of the CFS epidemic must be halted immediately. Congress must be spurred into action, to investigate what, I believe, is a cover-up of the extent and impact of this epidemic, and to appropriate many more millions of dollars for research.

You can make that happen. Every person who reads this book has the power to lobby elected officials, on all levels of government, to make CFS research the number-one public health priority.

If CFS does not become the number-one public health priority in the United States, the nation could become crippled, financially and in every other way, as more and more people are disabled by this illness.

50 THINGS YOU SHOULD KNOW ABOUT THE CHRONIC FATIGUE SYNDROME EPIDEMIC

1 CFS Often Begins Like The Flu

Chronic Fatigue Syndrome (CFS) is, right now, almost impossible to diagnose when it first begins, because it often appears to be identical to the flu. That's one reason why the official government definition requires that a person has to have been sick for more than six months to qualify for a diagnosis of CFS. With the development of more sophisticated laboratory tests, and the identification of what causes it, most researchers believe that problem will be resolved.

CFS usually begins with the onset of fever, fatigue, muscle and joint pain, headache, depression, sleep disturbance, painful lymph glands, and sore throat.

When the first known outbreak of CFS in the U.S. occurred in late 1984 and early 1985, the two physicians who described it thought their patients simply had a lingering flu. Dr. Daniel Peterson and Dr. Paul Cheney became concerned, however, when their patients in Incline Village, Nevada (near Lake Tahoe) didn't seem to be able to recover from their strange "flu." Drs. Cheney and Peterson became so concerned, in fact, that they called in the nation's experts on epidemics, the Centers for Disease Control (CDC).

The CDC investigators didn't take the Incline Village outbreak very seriously, which established an indifferent attitude to CFS that still lingers at that government research facility. Although CDC officials were aware of CFS from the time of that first outbreak, it wasn't until three years later, in early 1988, that they officially recognized the illness and gave it the name "Chronic Fatigue Syndrome."

As Cheney and Peterson soon discovered (even though the government researchers couldn't seem to figure it out), CFS is much more serious than the flu. People with CFS don't get better after a week or so; some symptoms can become dramatically worse over time.

Short-term memory loss can become so severe that a person is unable to watch television or read a book—he or she can't remember the plot of the story. Dizziness, depth perception, and balance problems can make it difficult for a CFS patient even to walk.

The eyes, as part of the central nervous system, can be severely affected by CFS. Patients often develop "floaters," little specks that float in the liquid inside the eye and interfere with vision. People with CFS can have trouble focusing their eyes; some have even developed an eye infection called "uveitis," which can result in a detached retina, leading to blindness.

Almost all CFS patients suffer from headaches and an increased sensitivity to sunlight and other forms of light. A small percentage (estimated at two or three percent) actually develop transient blindness (which comes and goes).

Seizures have been seen in a small number of CFS patients.

Sometimes CFS patients will feel better for a few days and then, usually for unknown reasons, the symptoms return.

The cyclic nature of these symptoms is one of CFS's most frustrating aspects, because it becomes impossible for patients to make plans or live any sort of a normal life. CFS patients can appear to be reasonably healthy one day, and they're suddenly bedridden the next.

Because CFS was first identified in people who had the financial resources to pursue medical treatment after they had been told by more than one physician that there was nothing wrong with them, CFS has been mostly mocked by the press, and given derisive names like "Yuppie Flu." Over the last six years, however, it has been demonstrated that CFS can strike anyone without warning: young and old, male and female, people of all races and across all economic classes.

But increasingly sophisticated measurements of immune system functioning is showing that CFS is actually an immune system disease. In fact, a June 1990 research report concluded that "CFS is a form of acquired immunodeficiency."

2 CFS Is Not Chronic Fatigue

One of the biggest drawbacks to the name "Chronic Fatigue Syndrome" is that the syndrome—a collection of many symptoms—can become confused with a single symptom: being chronically fatigued.

Why is that a problem? Fatigue, as any physician will tell you, is the symptom that patients report most often. People with a cold or the flu are tired; people with cancer are tired. People under stress, or working too hard, women who are pregnant or with new babies—all of these conditions can lead to chronic fatigue.

And, perhaps most unfortunately for people who have CFS, fatigue is one of the most prominent symptoms of depression. If a patient appears to be otherwise healthy, but goes to a doctor complaining of being tired all the time, one of the first things the doctor will suspect is that the patient is depressed. And, often, the doctor will be correct.

Chronic Fatigue *Syndrome* is a completely separate entity from chronic fatigue. But some researchers who don't believe that CFS exists have exploited this semantic confusion to try to prove that as high as 90 percent of people with CFS actually suffer from depression. And the popular press—which is unaccustomed to researchers twisting facts and figures to prove whether an illness exists—has regularly fallen into the trap of the confusion created by the term "chronic fatigue."

People with CFS are fatigued, certainly. But they describe their fatigue as being far beyond any sort of tiredness that they have ever experienced. It is so profound a fatigue that they often can't even find the words to describe it. One patient told me that his fatigue was so great that he could imagine just lying in bed for the rest of his life, watching the years pass him by, until he died. That's how severe—and how frightening—the fatigue is.

People with CFS, under the definition from the Centers for Disease Control in 1988, are required to have experienced fatigue so severe that it has lasted six months and that it has decreased their daily activities by half.

That would seem enough to most people to accept CFS as a serious illness. But other physiological and psychological illnesses also can cause severe and prolonged fatigue.

CFS has a variety of other symptoms that accompany the fatigue; these symptoms can be unremitting, or occur in cycles, waxing and waning. A patient may feel better for a few days or weeks, only to be suddenly struck down by a whole constellation of symptoms—including incapacitating fatigue—without warning.

3 CFS Is An Illness Of Immune Dysfunction

With Chronic Fatigue Syndrome, the patient's immune system doesn't work the way it should—it is dysfunctional. Why is that? It is believed that some kind of infectious agent—probably a virus—infects people with CFS and disrupts the normal functioning of the immune system. This could happen because the virus is killing the immune system cells, or because it disrupts one of the signals that tells the immune system cells when to reproduce themselves and what to attack. Right now, there is still a great deal of debate and controversy about what is causing the dysfunction.

But laboratory tests increasingly are showing that people with CFS have moderate to severe immune dysfunction, and that's why some patients and physicians favor changing the syndrome's name to "Chronic Fatigue Immune Dysfunction Syndrome," or CFIDS (pronounced See-fids). The *Atlanta Journal Constitution* reported that Dr. Walter Gunn, who is in charge of investigating the CFS epidemic at the Centers for Disease Control, said that the agency was even considering changing the name of the epidemic to Chronic Immune Dysfunction Syndrome.

Initially, the studies performed on CFS patients didn't show a clear pattern of immune dysfunction: In some people, certain parts of the immune system were more active; in others, less active. So it took scientists a while to figure out what kind of pattern to look for to help them diagnose CFS.

A physician in Manhattan, Dr. Ronald Hoffman, explains the pattern of immune dysfunction like this: Imagine that the immune system is a television set, and somebody walks over to the TV and gives it a good whack with a baseball bat. The TV would probably become dysfunctional, but how? Well, you might see vertical disruption of the picture; you might lose horizontal control; you could lose the sound, or the picture—or both—altogether. No two TV sets would respond exactly the same way, but the functioning of each would probably be disrupted.

The human immune system, of course, is far more complex than a TV, which makes it at the same time extremely vulnerable and incredibly adaptable. The adaptability allows the immune system to defend against many types of invaders: bacteria, viruses, and funguses. But if the delicate balance maintained by all the components of the immune system is sufficiently disturbed, the immune system can stop working, or can even attack the body itself. When the immune system becomes confused and attacks the body, an "autoimmune" disease—like lupus or arthritis—can develop.

Precisely how the human immune system works is a mystery which is continually being unraveled. Over the last few years, scientists have learned a great deal about various components of the immune system and how they interact.

One very important type of immune system cell is a subset of white cells called B-cells. B-cells produce antibodies that protect against disease; when a person has antibodies against a particular disease, such as smallpox, the person is said to be immunized.

When B-cells malfunction, however, they can go haywire and produce antibodies against invaders that are not really present; dysfunctional B-cells themselves can cause disease, even cancer.

Another group of white cells important to the immune system is the T-cells (now often called CD cells). There are many different types of T-cells. There are "helper" T-cells (T4 or CD4 cells) that "help" the B-cells turn on to produce antibodies. One type of T8 (CD8) cell is the "suppressor" CD8 cells that tell the immune system when to shut down.

It is very important to maintain a balance between the helper and suppressor cells so that the immune system knows not only when to go into action, but when to stop, as well. In people with

21

CFS, there is often an imbalance between these two types of cells, which means that the immune system does not respond appropriately to invaders.

Another very important—perhaps crucial—type of T-cell is called the "natural killer" (NK) cell. NK cells function as non-specific scavengers in the immune system, gobbling up cells that are infected by viruses and cancer cells. But in people with CFS, the NK cells don't function properly, which may be why CFS patients apparently develop cancers more often than the general population. If a cancer starts to grow, and the NK cells don't stop it right away, it can develop into a full-fledged malignancy.

Another group of immune system cells, the "phagocytic" cells, are capable of engulfing and destroying foreign matter (or defective cells). In the circulating blood, these cells are called monocytes; when they migrate to organ tissue (like lung and liver), they become macrophages. The phagocytic cells are very important in defending the body against invaders.

The phagocytic cells (as well as other white blood cells) produce substances called "cytokines" that help the various cells communicate with each other so that they know what to do. People with CFS can produce too few—or too many—of these substances; when cytokine production is disturbed, the immune system doesn't know when to turn on—or when to shut down.

As you can see by even this very simplistic description, the interactions of the various components of the immune system are very complex indeed. The miracle is that, in most people, the immune system functions almost perfectly most of the time.

But when a person develops CFS, the checks and balances within the healthy immune system are disrupted. The cells don't communicate properly with each other, and they don't know how to respond appropriately to invaders.

That's why CFS is best described as an illness of immune dysfunction.

4 CFS Is Not Depression

All too often, when a patient with undiagnosed CFS goes to a doctor to find out what is wrong, the patient will be told that he or she has depression. Although people with CFS may become unhappy or depressed because they are unable to work or lead a normal life, "depression" is a clinical entity that is completely separate from CFS.

Depression does not cause any of the physical symptoms—sore throat, swollen glands, fever, muscle aches—seen in CFS. And depression also does not cause the astounding, AIDS-like immunological abnormalities identified in people with CFS.

People who are depressed generally withdraw from life, lose enthusiasm, and don't care much about anything. But people with CFS are generally anxious to get back to work, very much engaged with trying to find a treatment for their illness, and care a great deal about rejoining society as healthy participants.

So why do many physicians still believe that CFS is a type of depression?

Some believe that theory has been fueled by research by one of the government's highest-ranking CFS researchers, Dr. Stephen Straus at the National Institute of Allergy and Infectious Diseases. As recently as January 1989, Dr. Straus and co-workers published a scientific article purporting to find a "lifetime history" of psychiatric illness among CFS patients—even though such a history is among the conditions that must be eliminated before a diagnosis of CFS can be given.

Many people who have studied the Chronic Fatigue Syndrome epidemic believe that the government does not want the American public to know how serious and widespread the problem is.

5 CFS Is A Contagious Illness

Research is increasingly showing that CFS is a contagious illness; that is, an illness which can be spread from one person to another, in an as-yet-unknown manner.

CFS has occurred in "epidemic outbreaks" since it was first identified. During the first outbreak in Incline Village, Nevada in 1984-85, 200 people in that small town became ill around the same time. While some local business people claimed the illness was due to a mass hysteria, Dr. Paul Cheney and Dr. Daniel Peterson, the two physicians investigating the outbreak, believed that an infectious agent—a virus or bacteria—was causing the illness.

In Lyndonville, New York, Dr. David Bell has been studying a "cluster outbreak" of CFS in which a number of the patients are children. Dr. Bell has found that half of the children have *at least* one other immediate family member who also developed CFS.

One of the most studied cases of an "epidemic outbreak" of CFS occurred in a symphony orchestra in the South. Dr. Ronald Herberman (at the University of Pittsburgh) studied this outbreak, in which eight out of 64 young, previously healthy people developed CFS at the same time—that's 12 percent of the orchestra.

Another outbreak of epidemic CFS studied by Dr. Herberman occurred among teachers in an elementary school in Ohio, in which seven teachers developed CFS during one year.

Since 1984, recognized clusters of CFS have occurred in Nevada, Pennsylvania, North Carolina, and New York.

Outbreaks have occurred in other parts of the world, as well. An outbreak of CFS in a hospital in Japan was studied by Dr. Herberman and a Japanese immunologist, Dr. Tadao Aoki (at the Shinrakuen Hospital in Niigata, Japan).

And in Canada, *Montreal Gazette* science editor Nicholas Regush has described how CFS moved through communities along the St. Lawrence River.

6 Pets Seem To Be Able To Catch CFS

For a number of years, people with CFS have suspected that their pets—dogs, cats, even horses—were coming down with CFS, too.

Does that sound crazy? Maybe it does. But there are a lot of illnesses that are transmitted from animals to people (although transmission in the other direction—from people to animals—is less well-documented).

Rabies, for instance, is a viral illness that infected animals can give to people. "Cat-scratch fever" is another such illness. There is even a bird illness, a lung infection called psitticosis, that humans can catch from domesticated birds like parrots.

Until recently, the only evidence that animals might be catching CFS had been largely "anecdotal"—literally, "stories" about such occurrences.

In 1990, however, Dr. Paul Cheney conducted a survey of people with CFS to find out if their pets really were getting sick much more often with unusual diseases. His office in Charlotte, North Carolina, gave questionnaires about pet illnesses to 68 consecutively seen, first-time patients with CFS who had pets.

What Dr. Cheney's survey showed was astonishing: Half of the CFS patients who responded to the questionnaire survey reported a severe or unusual illness in a pet. Among patients who didn't return the questionnaire, a survey of medical records revealed that almost 45 percent had reported the illness of a pet in their first interview at Dr. Cheney's office.

Of the 15 sick animals reported by Dr. Cheney's CFS patients, there were eight dogs (three of whom died) and seven cats (four of whom died). Four of the animals (two dogs, two cats) died of seizure or limb paralysis. One dog and one cat died of what Dr. Cheney called "abrupt undefined illness." And one cat died after an infected wound did not respond to antibiotics.

Five of the seven pet deaths occurred in pets who got sick at the same time as the CFS patient; one pet who died got sick before the patient, and one after.

Dr. Cheney divided the pet illnesses into five categories: 1. a

"CFS-like" illness with fevers, lethargy, allergies, and congestion (five animals); 2. a nervous system-type illness with limb paralysis, seizures, and loss of muscular coordination (four animals, which all died); 3. the "acute undefined illness" (three animals, two of which died); 4. a digestive illness with chronic or acute vomiting and diarrhea (two animals, one of which died); and 5. one animal which had only "allergies."

Are pets catching CFS from people? Or are the pets and the patients developing similar infections at around the same time from a third source?

Those questions remain unanswered, but until the situation is clarified, Dr. Cheney advises his patients not to share food scraps with their pets—just in case.

7 Children Can Catch CFS

Dr. David Bell is one of the few physicians in the U.S. who has studied CFS in children. Dr. Bell practices in Lyndonville, New York, where an outbreak of epidemic CFS occurred: Over a two-year period (1985-1987), two hundred people in the small town of Lyndonville became ill with CFS. (After the CDC criteria for CFS were established, it was found that 104 of these patients met the criteria.) Dr. Bell recently discussed a study of 18 children who became sick with CFS during the Lyndonville outbreak.

Dr. Bell believes that, while children may experience more symptoms which are different from adults, they have essentially the same illness—that is, CFS *does* strike children.

In all, thirty-six children were part of the Lyndonville outbreak, and half of these children had at least one other family member who was also sick. This situation is called a "family cluster," and Dr. Bell points out that such family clusters of CFS have been reported *all over the world*.

In earlier studies, Dr. Bell's research showed that the children with CFS have immune systems that are disturbed in much the same way as adult patients' immune systems.

26

For example, natural killer cell activity was lowered in the children, as it is in adults. The children also had disturbed T4/T8 cell ratios. And they were unable to respond to immunologic skin tests, like adults with CFS.

Some of the children had elevated levels of antibodies to Human Herpesvirus 6 (HHV-6), but Dr. Bell points out that the "normal" levels of antibodies to this virus in children have never been determined.

The children in Dr. Bell's most recent study came from only nine families. Two families each had four sick children; two other families each had two sick children. The other families had one sick child each.

These children became sick at around the same time, and all had essentially the same symptoms. Eleven of them had what Dr. Bell calls "acute onset" (getting very sick quite suddenly), and seven had "gradual onset." Twelve were male; six, female. Each child had been sick for three to four years at the time of Dr. Bell's study.

They all had fatigue, headache and nervous system disorders, joint pain, abdominal pain, and recurrent sore throat. Seventeen of the children also had lymph node tenderness and muscle pain. Other symptoms common among them were rashes, fevers, and chills.

Dr. Bell believes that children with CFS have a pretty good chance of getting better, at least partially, over time. When these children first became sick, they were all severely ill; some actually became bedridden.

Four years later, however, most of the children were able to resume about 75 percent of their activities, with only mild or moderate symptoms. Only a few patients still had a more than 50 percent reduction in activity (necessary to meet the CDC criteria).

"None of the children in the study consider themselves free of whatever is the disease process we're calling CFIDS, and that's somewhat alarming," Dr. Bell said of these children. "However, their improvement in terms of activity and symptoms has been significant."

8 Anyone Can Catch CFS

Anyone can catch CFS, "including children," according to Ottawa physician Dr. Byron Hyde, "after contact with a person coughing in the elevator or in the next aircraft seat," as Dr. Hyde told *Montreal Gazette* science editor Nicholas Regush.

But who is at most risk for catching CFS?

Dr. Hyde thinks that "those people with increased public exposure, such as teachers, doctors, nurses, airline stewardesses, are the most vulnerable."

Outbreaks have been documented among school teachers, high school sports teams, hospital workers, and a symphony orchestra, in addition to entire families and communities.

Health care workers may be especially vulnerable to CFS. In spring 1987, a physician wrote a letter to then-Surgeon General C. Everett Koop to warn him about the potential danger that CFS (then called "Chronic Epstein-Barr Virus" [CEBV] Syndrome) posed to the military. This letter was released to me under a Freedom of Information Act request, and I'd like you to read some of what it said.

"I am a middle-aged board-certified physician and have had the misfortune of contracting 'chronic Epstein-Barr virus reactivation syndrome' ('chronic mononucleosis' or 'CEBV') four years ago," this doctor wrote. "I had had a productive, satisfying, medical practice prior to that time and had been in excellent health, but awoke with a severe sore throat and flu-like illness one day and have been totally disabled since, solely due to 'CEBV.' "

The physician expressed some very grave concerns to Surgeon General Koop.

"This letter concerns chronic mononucleosis and the possibility that the contagious but unidentified-as-yet virus causing it is also the trigger for full-blown AIDS," the physician wrote in early 1987. "I *personally* know many (about 40) health care workers who have contracted CEBV since 1981, all of whom were previously healthy, and all of whom worked with AIDS or lymphoma patients, usually through working in intensive care unit direct patient care, or as oncology nurses, or as ear-nose-throat doctors at the time they became ill. I am writing about a highly contagious, rapidly spreading, viral epidemic in America now occurring that is a more serious threat to our society than AIDS.''

This physician was particularly concerned about CFS's threat to the armed services. The italics are his.

"I have already been told of the occurrence of *total disability* due to CEBV recently requiring some soldiers to leave the service," he wrote. "The CEBV epidemic could have a disastrous effect on our armed services, much more dangerous than AIDS, due to its ability to *rapidly spread like the common cold*. Since it can spread as quickly as it recently did in Lake Tahoe, where over 500 people contracted it within several months, it can *quickly disable entire bases*, as well as leave a large number of permanently disabled at great expense."

The physician urged the Surgeon General to use his influence to demand that several senior investigators at the major health agencies—the Centers for Disease Control and the National Institutes of Health—devote all their efforts to identifying the cause of the CFS epidemic.

"Powers similar to that of a General in war time should be given to these senior officials," the physician suggested.

Although Surgeon General Koop received this letter in early 1987, the "activist Surgeon General"—like the rest of the U.S. government health apparatus—did nothing.

And more than four years later, most of the questions raised by this physician remain unanswered—including the question of who is at most risk for developing CFS.

9 CFS Is Potentially A Major Problem For Airline Safety

People in the airline industry may be at increased risk for developing CFS. Some experts believe that people who are in contact with the public on a daily basis—like teachers, health care workers, pilots, and flight attendants—may be at the greatest risk for developing the syndrome.

29

If that theory is true, pilots—upon whom thousands of people depend for safe transportation every day—may be one of the most important groups of CFS patients to identify.

A pilot who is also a physician has written about trying to fly a plane after he developed CFS.

As the doctor/pilot was attempting to land his plane one morning, using the routine flight plan he had followed for several years, he suddenly realized that he was on the wrong runway—but only because the control tower operator couldn't locate his plane.

The doctor/pilot realized that he couldn't remember which way was right—or left.

And he also realized, suddenly, that he'd had trouble remembering his flight plan throughout what was for him a very routine flight.

Miraculously, he landed safely—but only after the tower operator guided him through his landing, a procedure the doctor had been following on his own for more than 25 years.

And when the doctor/pilot flew the next time, he had increasingly severe problems remembering words, commands, and directions. He finally realized that the confusion he had been experiencing recently meant he was really sick.

The doctor/pilot had developed CFS. Two-and-a-half years previously, he came down with what he thought was the flu, with a low-grade fever, sore throat, muscle pain, headaches, and fatigue.

He got a little better, but when he tried to exercise, he had a severe relapse from which he never fully recovered. Like most CFS patients, the pilot—even though a physician himself—went to specialist after specialist, with no results.

Two years after he first became sick, the doctor's remittant symptoms became suddenly worse: He developed facial tics, sleeping difficulties, constant nightmares, night sweats, and severe muscle pains when he tried to exercise. Finally, he was forced to quit his job.

This doctor/pilot was very concerned that flight surgeons should be on the look-out for pilots who might have the syndrome.

He was especially concerned that pilots with undiagnosed CFS might be flying planes—and presenting a great risk to aviation safety.

Flight surgeons, especially, should learn the signs and symptoms of CFS; otherwise, an undetermined number of confused pilots, who are unable to remember their flight plans and distinguish right from left, may be flying—or crashing—airplanes.

10 CFS Is Pandemic— A World-Wide Epidemic

CFS is not just a health problem in the United States—it has also been detected in Japan, Canada, Germany, Great Britain, New Zealand, and Australia.

In Japan, scientists published a scientific report describing "Low Natural Killer Syndrome" (LNKS) in 1987. LNKS was characterized by "uncomfortable fatigue" and recurrent fever, lasting at least six months with no explanation. That description is strikingly similar to the description written the following year by the American scientists who created the case definition of CFS.

German Professor Gerhard Krueger (University of Cologne) said in late 1988 on a television show in the U.S. that, in then-West Germany, four out of every 1,000 patients seen in medical practices appeared to develop CFS. He compared that with the incidence of breast cancer, which is approximately 35 per 100,000 patients.

"I think AIDS is not such a serious problem as compared to the Chronic Fatigue Syndrome," Professor Krueger said.

In New Zealand, Dr. J.C. Murdoch studies CFS and in Britain—where it is called "myalgic encephalomyelitis"—the syndrome has been studied extensively by Dr. P.O. Behan.

In New South Wales, Australia, Dr. Andrew Lloyd (now working at the U.S. National Cancer Institute) performed an epidemiologic study in New South Wales to determine how widespread CFS is in that country. He discussed that study's findings at a research conference in the U.S. in early 1991.

Dr. Lloyd and his research team determined that approximately one out of every 3,000 people had the syndrome. These patients had been sick for an average of five to six years at the time of the study, which meant that they—like many patients in the U.S.—became ill around 1984.

In Canada, there are a "large number" of physicians who have CFS, according to Ottawa physician and researcher Dr. Byron Hyde. He has found that many CFS patients appear to be professional people—healthcare workers, teachers—who are in contact with a lot of people.

Doctors who treat the disease often end up getting it themselves, along with their wives and children.

The economic impact of CFS is enormous, Dr. Hyde believes; he estimates that $100 *billion* worth of salaries has been lost due to CFS in the United States and Canada alone.

Dr. Hyde announced at a conference in early 1991 that the Canadian government has agreed to fund health clinics in Canadian university centers so that CFS can be studied—and patients can receive treatment—in every province of the country.

"When your congress finds only $1 million for the CDC's epidemiologic study...I wonder where your congress's priorities are," Dr. Hyde told conference participants.

The U.S. Centers for Disease Control is currently conducting a "surveillance study" to attempt to estimate how many people in this country have CFS. Preliminary results from that study may be ready by late summer 1992. A November 12, 1990 cover story about CFS in *Newsweek*, however, quoted estimates from epidemiologists that two to five million Americans may already have the AIDS-like illness. Some researchers believe as many as ten million people in the U.S. may already have CFS.

Nobody knows how many cases of CFS exist in any country, but experts agree on one thing—CFS is attacking the immune systems of people all over the world.

11 The Press Has Ignored CFS— Or Made Fun Of It

The press, following the lead of U.S. health authorities, has not been kind to CFS patients. Indeed, the press has been extremely skeptical about CFS.

It is not just that the press has ignored the plight of CFS patients, many of whom lose their jobs, their marriages, their homes, their cars—and their health. In newspaper, television, and radio reports, CFS patients have been ridiculed for many years.

Some press reports have suggested that CFS is a form of depression, or another psychological illness. Some have hypothesized that people with CFS are hypochondriacs or malingerers, suggesting that CFS patients should just pull themselves together.

One of the most damaging things that the press has done is to confer the name "Yuppie Flu" on CFS. The "Yuppie Flu" is a product of stress experienced by over-achieving Yuppies, according to this press theory, the implication being that CFS is just the latest in a series of fad diagnoses and not a real illness at all.

The British press has been just as vicious as the American press. In England, CFS is called "myalgic encephalomyelitis," or ME. The British press has called ME "the 'me' disease."

12 People With CFS Are Unable To Exercise

One of the ways physicians who are knowledgeable about CFS diagnose it is the patient's response to exercising. People with CFS almost always suffer a relapse after attempting to exercise.

This unusual response to physical exercise is used by Dr. Paul Cheney as a diagnostic tool; he says that patients' decline after exercising can be dramatic.

Manhattan's Dr. Ronald Hoffman also uses exercise intolerance as a guide when diagnosing CFS.

"One of the most important manifestations is a person's response to exercising," Dr. Hoffman told me in an interview. "If

I'm not sure what's going on with a person, I say, 'You're kind of tired, you're under a lot of stress. Most people begin to feel better if they get on an exercise program. *I* feel better if I exercise. How do you feel when you exercise? If you ran around the reservoir, at your own pace, how would you feel?' If the patient says to me, 'I could maybe do it, but at the end of it, it would set me back so tremendously that I would probably have to stay in bed for a week,' that is very, very diagnostic of this syndrome. The will to do it is there, but they feel really wiped out afterward.''

Unfortunately, patients are often mistakenly told to exercise by doctors who think they are suffering from depression, and this bad recommendation can make a person with CFS much sicker.

I interviewed a patient named Susan (not her real name) whose doctor told her to "exercise her way into health." When she tried to follow his advice, she became very ill.

"Aerobics nearly killed me," Susan told me.

Even the Centers for Disease Control's case definition for CFS recognizes that exercise can make CFS patients worse. One of the criteria that patients must fulfill to be diagnosed with CFS is "prolonged fatigue after exercise."

No one knows why people with CFS have such a dramatic, negative response to exercising. Some evidence now suggests that people with CFS have an elevated heart rate, which can cause them to tire easily.

13 Miscarriage Is Common In CFS

Like many aspects of CFS, miscarriage is a rather mysterious complication not clearly understood, but which appears to be quite common in pregnant women with CFS.

Comedienne Gilda Radner had a miscarriage around the time she first developed symptoms of CFS (called "Chronic Epstein-Barr Virus," CEBV, syndrome at that time), and she wrote about it in her autobiography, *It's Always Something*.

Dr. Paul Cheney finds a "relatively high" incidence of miscarriage and low birth-weight babies among his pregnant patients. At a conference in early 1990, Cheney reported that, of the seven pregnant women he has treated for CFS, four miscarried. Of the three babies born, two were low birth-weight babies. Cheney described these babies as "small or skinny," but said they seemed to grow normally.

More disturbingly, however, Cheney said he had heard that one of the children born to a mother with CFS, at the age of nine months developed a series of bacterial infections, one of which was life-threatening.

Other reproductive system abnormalities appear to occur in CFS. One is endometriosis, a very painful condition in which the lining of the uterus migrates and grows elsewhere.

Dr. Perry Orens, a Long Island physician who has a large practice of people with CFS, told me in a recent interview, "There's unquestionably a hormonal factor in CFIDS [Chronic Fatigue Immune Dysfunction Syndrome, another name for CFS]."

"One of the questions that a physician asks a menstruating female is, what happens when you get your menstrual period?" Dr. Orens explained. "Almost always they [CFS patients] will tell you that their symptoms are exaggerated, they are worse. No matter how bad the symptoms generally are, they get worse during the woman's menstrual periods. And I don't think there's any question but that there's an enormous percentage of women who have endometriosis and CFIDS—it's way beyond the expected norms.

"So I think there is a hormonal factor involved, probably on a secondary basis," he continued. "I don't think that hormonal differences between men and women are the causes of CFIDS, but I think that CFIDS causes exaggerated changes in the female, and that's one reason why we see so much endometriosis in women with CFIDS."

I asked Dr. Orens if he knew of any virus that produces that kind of effect. He replied, "I know of no virus that does that—other than the one that is probably causing CFIDS."

14 Serious Heart Irregularities Can Develop In CFS

Certain types of heart abnormalities can develop in people with CFS. Primarily these abnormalities are disturbances in the rhythm and speed of the heartbeat, similar to what President George Bush suffered in spring 1991.

Dr. Paul Cheney has observed chest pain, several types of heartbeat irregularities, and heart murmurs in his CFS patients. He has even seen a few patients who developed an inflammation of a section of heart muscle.

Ten to 20 percent of Dr. Cheney's patients develop a particular kind of heart murmur called a "mitral valve prolapse." This type of heart murmur produces a distinctive clicking sound.

CFS patient "Susan" had a dog who got sick around the same time that she first developed symptoms of CFS. (There is speculation that pets can also catch CFS, and Susan believes that several of her pets have contracted the illness.)

The dog died of a rapid, irregular beating of the heart ("fibrillation"), a condition that can also kill people.

"I have a heart irregularity, too, but I can't get any of the doctors to give me a definite diagnosis," Susan told me.

Dr. Carol Jessup, who began studying CFS as an associate professor of medicine at the University of California (San Francisco) in 1983, now has a private practice in which she has seen more than 1,300 CFS patients. Although she finds low blood pressure in 86 percent of her CFS patients, she said at a November 1990 conference in Charlotte, North Carolina that she finds a rapid heartbeat in some patients.

Dr. Anthony Komaroff is a CFS researcher at the Boston Brigham and Women's Hospital. At a conference held in Pittsburgh in September 1988, Dr. Komaroff reported that as high as 40 to 50 percent of his CFS patients experience rapid heart rates.

Some researchers have speculated that a rapid heart rate may contribute to the extreme fatigue that CFS patients experience after exercising.

15 Digestive Problems Develop In CFS

Many people with CFS are plagued by digestive system problems—diarrhea, distended stomach, and stomach pain.

Why is this? It may be because of an overproduction of histamine, produced naturally by the body to control the production of stomach acids. When too much histamine floods the body, too much stomach acid can be produced, resulting in stomach distress.

One CFS patient I interviewed, "Al," developed severe diarrhea when he became ill with CFS. Because his doctor didn't know much about CFS, he told Al that he had "spastic colon," and referred him to a psychiatrist.

Partly because of these stomach problems, Al lost 55 pounds in one year.

Another hint that histamine may be involved in the stomach problems experienced by CFS patients is that they develop allergies; too much histamine is also produced in some types of allergies. After having CFS for nearly two years, Al suddenly developed new, severe allergies. When he was tested for sensitivity to 15 substances that produce allergic responses, he was sensitive to every single one.

"Susan" also developed severe diarrhea when she became ill with CFS. Her housemate developed chronic diarrhea and stomach cramps, as well.

Susan also has had two dogs who developed serious stomach problems: diarrhea and "projectile" vomiting. (As I have already pointed out, pets seem to be able to "catch" CFS and often have symptoms very similar to those of their sick owners.)

Susan told me that she, her friend, and her dog, "are sometimes all three taking the same stomach medication."

In some cases, digestive problems may actually be the first symptom of the syndrome. One doctor in California discovered that a majority of her CFS patients had digestive problems before they developed flu-like symptoms of Chronic Fatigue Syndrome.

16 CFS Can Cause Eye Disease— Even Blindness

The eyes are part of the central nervous system, connected directly to the brain. Therefore, many illnesses of the central nervous system can also affect the eyes.

Even though as high as four percent of people with CFS can develop transient blindness (a non-permanent blindness), the illness's effect on eyes has not been a focus of many studies. However, Dr. David J. Browning, an associate of Dr. Paul Cheney and an eye surgeon, has studied how CFS affects the eyes.

The most common eye problems are extreme light sensitivity, "floaters," occasional double vision or blurring of vision, and burning and pain in the eyes.

"Floaters" are specks that float in the patient's field of vision and move as the eye moves, according to Dr. Browning. They generally are clumps of collagen and although floaters usually aren't serious, they can signal serious eye disease (such as a torn retina or inflammation). There is no treatment for floaters.

Eye fatigue is probably responsible for the blurring of vision that CFS patients experience. When someone is very fatigued, he or she may not have the energy to make the eyes work together as they normally do.

Dr. Browning also notes that medications that affect the central nervous system, like anti-depressants, can make the problem of blurred vision worse.

Double vision has the same source in CFS patients—not enough energy to coordinate the focus of the two eyes. Both double and blurred vision should be treated with rest, Dr. Browning advises.

The extreme light sensitivity experienced by CFS patients is a mystery to Dr. Browning, he admits. He advises people with light sensitivity to wear sunglasses that can block the sun's rays.

Pain and burning in the eye is often caused by "dry eye," in which not enough tears are produced to lubricate the eye's motion. Dr. Browning suggests tear replacement (with artificial tears) and, occasionally, oral tetracycline (an antibiotic) if an eye infection is suspected.

A very small number of CFS patients can develop serious eye infections, often related to a viral infection, which can reduce vision to the point of legal blindness. For these types of infections, Dr. Browning recommends treatment with an antiviral drug called Acyclovir.

Another condition that can threaten vision in CFS patients is the new growth of blood vessels beneath the retina, which lines the back of the eye. This very serious condition can be treated by a therapy (using laser beams) which destroys the new vessels.

17 CFS Patients Have Trouble Thinking Clearly

Al, a CFS patient in Brooklyn, knew he was seriously ill when he started having trouble making change in his job as bartender. "It wasn't just my blurry vision—I already had trouble focusing at that time—but I was having problems, too, with adding and subtracting," said Al.

And, over the five years he has been sick, Al's mental problems have worsened.

"I used to keep a journal, and now when I go back and read it, I can't understand the words that I once wrote," Al told me. "I can't begin to express thoughts in writing. There are times when I can't read at all—it makes no sense—it's like reading Greek. I have actually had to look up the word 'of' because I can't remember what it means."

Al says he feels like he has a "fogginess in the brain" which makes it a struggle to think or read. Many CFS patients have described this "fogginess" to me, using exactly the same images.

Al even has had periods of amnesia during which he can't remember where he is or what he is doing.

Another CFS patient, "David," also described his mental problems to me. He has experienced a bizarre, haunting feeling like "a decay in the brain, like it was actually rotting away," he told me. "I couldn't focus on anything during these periods" when he had this feeling, David says.

At other times, David has a disoriented feeling "like being in a pea soup"; he is then afraid to stand or walk.

"Marie" is a patient in California, who spent three months completely disabled because her brain was in a constant state of seizure. Even after the seizures were controlled with medication, Marie had very serious mental problems. She couldn't concentrate well enough to read or watch television. And she found that, when she tried to write, her hand would soar uncontrollably up the page.

Many CFS patients have similar—if not always so severe—intellectual problems, most notably memory loss.

18 People With CFS Have Unusual Brain Waves

One of the ways that scientists can measure if a person's brain is working properly is by examining the electrical activity it generates. There are four distinct patterns of electrical activity produced; these patterns are called brain waves.

Brain waves are measured by electroencephalogram, or EEG. An abnormal EEG tells a physician that something is malfunctioning in the brain's electrical system.

The four types of brain waves are named after letters in the Greek alphabet: alpha (a state of calm or relaxation), beta (in which intellectual functioning occurs), theta (the state of drowsiness before falling asleep), and delta (the brain wave seen during deep sleep).

A researcher in Charlotte, North Carolina, Myra Preston, is studying the brain waves of CFS patients. What she has discovered is shocking: The brain wave pattern seen in CFS patients is exactly the opposite of the brain wave pattern of healthy people.

When a healthy person is awake and functioning, Ms. Preston explained to me, the brain produces primarily a combination of alpha and beta waves.

But CFS patients produce very low levels of alpha and beta brain waves.

Instead, CFS patients seem to be "stuck" in theta—their brains produce high levels of the brain wave associated with drowsiness, even when they are awake.

The result, Ms. Preston explains, is that CFS patients are never fully awake and able to function intellectually; neither can they fall deeply asleep.

Ms. Preston has studied 80 CFS patients, and found that 95 percent of them produced this type of abnormal brain wave.

People with CFS sometimes have dramatic drops in IQ measurements; some patients have been reported to lose 30 IQ points after they develop CFS. And CFS patients also report that they have trouble sleeping, which contributes to their fatigue.

The abnormal brain wave pattern that Ms. Preston has detected may help explain the intellectual problems—like memory loss— and sleep disturbance that CFS patients experience.

Similar types of brain malfunction can be caused by viruses, according to Ms. Preston, and it is possible that the same virus that is attacking the immune systems of CFS patients is also attacking the central nervous system.

19 The Brain Cannot Get Enough Sugar To Function In CFS

A new type of brain scan, called a "PET scan," measures the rate of sugar usage in the brain. Dr. Steven Lottenberg, a physician at the University of California-Irvine, discussed how sugar usage is disturbed in the brains of people with CFS at a recent research conference.

Abnormal brain function is often associated with a physical abnormality. Physical changes in the brain can be seen using a type of brain scan called MRI. Using MRI and PET scans together can pinpoint the area of the brain that is not working properly and provide clues as to why.

After giving patients a specially-labeled sugar, there is a 32-35 minute period of increased sugar uptake in the brain during which abnormalities can be detected. After this period, sugar uptake returns to its usual rate. Dr. Lottenberg studied a small group of

CFS patients, four women and two men, and compared the sugar uptake in their brains to a similar group of healthy individuals.

In four regions of the brain—including the area in the front of the brain which governs thinking or cognition—CFS patients had very decreased glucose uptake, Dr. Lottenberg discovered.

Although this is a very sophisticated—and currently very expensive—research tool unavailable to most physicians, it may provide valuable clues to why CFS patients can't concentrate or remember.

20 CFS Disrupts The Electrical Activity Of The Brain

CFS often disrupts patients' ability to think clearly and form the memories necessary for learning. Dr. Marshall J. Handleman has studied the memory and learning problems in people with CFS, by using a brain mapping system, called BEAM, at the University of Southern California School of Medicine.

At a recent scientific conference, Dr. Handleman explained that certain behaviors can be "mapped" to certain areas of the brain; if an injury occurs in a particular section of the brain, very specific behaviors can become impaired.

The areas of the brain that are responsible for complex tasks like language, thought, judgment, attention, and physical coordination have only recently been identified, Dr. Handleman pointed out.

Dr. Handleman believes that much of the cognitive dysfunction seen in CFS patients results from their inability to make memories, both visual and auditory, and to turn short-term memories into long-term memories. Long-term memory is believed to be stored in a different portion of the brain from short-term memory.

The long-term memories formed before people became ill with CFS are not disturbed by the illness, Dr. Handleman stated; the CFS patient is simply unable to place new information into long-term memory.

42

And although people with CFS retain the long-term memory that they had before becoming ill, Dr. Handleman pointed out that they may have more trouble retrieving it.

He also has documented a variety of mental abnormalities in CFS patients using a system which measures the electrical activity in the brain.

In addition to memory disturbance, people with CFS can develop a condition in which numbers or letters are reversed: Seeing "54" instead of "45," as an example.

People with CFS often develop problems using language, like using the wrong word, being unable to remember the correct word to use, and having difficulty learning new languages. Dr. Handleman also noted that CFS patients have trouble with arithmetic.

Memory, mood, drive, and motivation can be impaired in CFS patients, Dr. Handleman said, and all of these functions are controlled by the same area of the brain. He speculated that there might be a virus infecting this area of the brain.

21 Blood Flow In The Brain Is Disrupted In CFS

The continuity of blood flow within the brain can now be measured by using a technology called "SPECT." It is relatively inexpensive because it uses radioactive substances used commonly in medicine. Dr. Ismael Mena, a professor of radiology at the University of California-Los Angeles, has studied brain blood flow in CFS patients.

Two radioactive substances can be used in SPECT scanning, Dr. Mena explained; one is inhaled, and the other is injected, but both cross the blood-brain barrier (the natural defense that keeps viruses, chemicals, and other invaders away from the brain).

The radioactive gas is inhaled, Dr. Mena stated, and then the brain is examined to see how fast the gas disappears. If it disappears quickly, blood flow is increased; if it disappears slowly, however, the blood flow is decreased.

Dr. Mena discussed two CFS patients who had received the

radioactive gas and then undergone SPECT scans. Both had a blood flow that was half as much as it should be.

Dr. Mena also discussed a study he had performed on 46 CFS patients. All patients were injected with a radioactive substance which would permeate the spaces in the brain. The patients were found to have diminished blood flow in four areas of the brain, including the area that governs thinking and learning.

Dr. Mena explained that there is normally a difference in the blood flow in the right and left sides of the brain. In the CFS patients, however, that difference was twice as much as normal.

If there is not enough blood flowing through the brain, not enough oxygen is being delivered to allow the brain to function normally.

22 There Is A CFS Dementia

Dr. Carl Sandman has studied the abnormal thinking and reasoning in CFS patients which he calls a "CFS dementia." Dr. Sandman is Chief of Research at the California Developmental Research Institute (in Cosa Mesa).

Using a variety of tests, Dr. Sandman studied 39 CFS patients and concluded that there is a distinct pattern of dysfunctional thought associated with the syndrome.

CFS patients are particularly poor at assembling puzzles, one of the tests performed by Dr. Sandman. Dr. Sandman hypothesized that CFS patients are distracted by any extra information in their environments.

"I've seen patients close an eye to solve the test, cock their heads in a funny way, posture themselves in some funny ways—strategies that they've learned to use to minimize distraction," Dr. Sandman pointed out at a scientific conference in February 1990.

There is a very distinct pattern to the mental difficulties that CFS patients exhibit, Dr. Sandman found. First, CFS patients have difficulty making memories. Once a memory is made, they can recall it; the difficulty lies in making the memory in the first place.

Second, people with CFS cannot overcome interference with memories—if they are distracted while trying to remember something, like a series of numbers, they lose the memory. Normally, this type of interference does not inhibit memory.

Third, CFS patients perform tasks like putting a puzzle together more slowly than healthy people because they can't think fast enough.

23 People With CFS Can Develop Brain Lesions

One of the most disturbing findings about CFS is that patients can develop brain lesions. Lesions are areas of abnormal tissue which can be detected by a variety of methods. Although it has not been proven what symptoms these lesions cause in CFS patients, they are clear-cut evidence of organic (physical) brain disease—which is extremely serious all by itself.

The first documented outbreak of CFS occurred in Lake Tahoe, Nevada, in late 1984 and early 1985. One of the physicians who identified that first outbreak, Dr. Paul Cheney, has continued to follow the patients involved. He has described the lesions he found at that time in the Lake Tahoe patients.

Dr. Cheney has shown, using types of tests that "map" nervous system problems to sites in the brain where there is physical damage, that the brains of people with CFS have been damaged.

Using a special kind of brain scan, Dr. Cheney discovered lesions in the brains of some Lake Tahoe patients. He also found that more of the patients who had been sick the longest (prior to 1986) showed abnormalities on brain scans than did those who had been sick for a shorter period of time.

Dr. Cheney also discovered that brain lesion development appeared to be age-dependent. Fifty percent of the Lake Tahoe teenagers involved in the epidemic had developed brain lesions by 1988; 33 percent of patients in their 20s, 35 percent of patients in their 30s, and 52 percent of patients in their 40s had developed brain lesions. In patients past the age of 50, Dr. Cheney found that 78 percent had developed brain lesions.

In early 1990, Dr. Cheney discussed new findings on the development of brain lesions in the Lake Tahoe patients: Two patients with brain lesions developed a rare cancer (called B-cell lymphoma) of the salivary gland.

Dr. Cheney also examined the cases of two school teachers involved in the epidemic. One of the teachers had no brain lesions the first time she had a brain scan. But when she had a scan later, she had developed a lesion.

In fact, 83 percent of the 60 patients from the Lake Tahoe epidemic had developed brain lesions by February 1990.

Dr. Cheney also examined "contact controls"—people not involved in the Lake Tahoe epidemic but in contact with people who were—with brain scans. He found, frighteningly, that 30 percent of the contact controls had also developed brain lesions.

24 CFS Patients Lose A Vital Part Of Their Immune Systems

Skin is very important in defending the body against invaders. Foreign agents—like viruses and bacteria—can enter the body when the skin is broken. If invaders can be stopped at the border (the skin), often they can be repelled altogether. So invaders must be identified accurately at the skin to stop them from going throughout the body.

In CFS patients, however, a very important part of the immune system appears to be lost: the recognition of foreign agents, called antigens, on the skin.

The skin of many CFS patients basically loses its intelligence.

The process that identifies antigens at the level of skin is called "cell-mediated immunity," because it is governed by immune system cells called T-cells.

Dr. J.C. Murdoch, a CFS researcher in Dunedin, New Zealand, has studied cell-mediated immunity in CFS patients. He compared the test results from the CFS patients with test results from an equal number of healthy individuals.

Cell-mediated immunity is measured by a type of skin test in which common antigens are injected into the skin. If the immune system is intact and can identify the antigens, a reaction (a raised, hard bump) will occur. If the immune system has been damaged, however, no response will be seen.

Dr. Murdoch tested the CFS patients against seven common antigens: tetanus, diphtheria, streptococcus, tuberculin, candida, trichophyton, and protease. Anyone with a healthy immune system would be expected to respond to these antigens. He found that there was a big difference between CFS patients' skin test results and those from the healthy patients.

In 1988, this lack of cell-mediated immunity prompted Dr. Murdoch to hypothesize that the syndrome "may be the result of acquired immune deficiency."

Dr. Nancy Klimas (at the University of Miami) also found, in a very detailed study of the immune systems of people with CFS, that cell-mediated immunity was lowered in 80 percent of the patients she studied. Dr. Klimas discovered that the CFS patients' test results were comparable to those she observed in a group of drug users infected with HIV (the so-called AIDS virus).

In 1990, Dr. Klimas wrote that her findings "suggest that CFS is a form of acquired immunodeficiency."

25 Skin Problems Can Develop In CFS

One aspect of CFS that puzzles physicians and scientists is the number of organs that can be affected by the illness. Although we don't usually think of our skin as being an organ, it does protect us from infections. When the skin is broken or ulcerated, bacteria and other infectious agents have a door into the body opened for them.

Rashes can develop in people who have CFS; Dr. David Bell, who studies CFS in children in upstate New York, has found that rashes are very common in children.

There is an illness of fever and rash seen in infants called "Roseola" that is now thought to be caused by Human Herpes Virus 6 (HHV-6). Herpes viruses are known to be capable of causing ulcerations like cold sores. People with CFS have elevated levels of antibodies to HHV-6.

Dr. Paul Cheney has found that CFS patients often develop blisters and ulcerations in the tissue that lines the mouth. They can also develop an oral infection called "thrush" (a common infection among AIDS patients) caused by an overgrowth of a common yeast.

CFS patients sometimes develop tumors, as "Susan" has. Susan has a tumor on her side, a few inches above her waist.

"It started out the size of a pea," Susan told me, "but now [in December 1990] it has grown to be about the size of a fingertip."

Susan has other skin problems. The worst skin problem she has is that the skin "peels off" her hands; it is very painful and debilitating.

"Maria," another CFS patient, has bleeding under the skin of one of her eyes, which creates a "spiderweb" appearance. The bleeding seems to be aggravated by warm water, exposure to sunlight, or mental exertion like trying to read or write during a headache. She told me that a severe headache by itself can cause the bleeding under her eye to occur.

Is a virus causing these various types of skin problems? Viruses certainly can cause rashes, tumors, and even bleeding (viruses that cause bleeding are called "hemorrhagic"). And if a virus is causing ulcerations, tumors, and bleeding on and under the skin, it is important to consider that the same conditions could be occurring inside the body as well.

26 People With CFS Can Lose Their Fingerprints

One of the most bizarre symptoms of CFS was discovered by Dr. Paul Cheney: CFS patients can lose their fingerprints.

"I keep talking about this, and as I've said before, I'll keep talking until someone tells me to shut up about it," Dr. Cheney said at a CFS conference in early 1990.

Dr. Cheney described the disappearance of the lines and ridges that create a distinct fingerprint. About 25 percent of his CFS patients lose their fingerprints.

Dr. Cheney has fingerprint cards made for all of his patients by local police.

"I always ask the patients to ask the deputy sheriffs who do the fingerprint cards if they've ever seen anything like this," Dr. Cheney said, "and the patients report that they always say no."

If CFS were to affect much of the general population, it would have serious implications for law enforcement.

27 Red Blood Cells Become Deformed In CFS

There are two main types of blood cells, red blood cells (RBCs) and white blood cells (WBCs). WBCs are primarily part of the immune system, although they have other functions—like helping to form blood clots—as well.

Red blood cells, however, carry oxygen all over the body. In order to deliver oxygen to every nook and cranny of the body's organs, RBCs must have very specific physical characteristics: They must be round, flexible enough to be able to change shape to slip through membranes, and strong enough not to break apart in the process. Rigid or malformed RBCs are unable to deliver the proper amount of oxygen to the body.

Researchers in New Zealand have studied the RBCs of people with CFS, and have found them to be defective. Dr. Leslie O. Simpson, one New Zealand researcher, has even suggested that the type of red cell abnormality observed could be used to help diagnose CFS.

Dr. Simpson examined the RBCs from people with CFS under a scanning electron microscope, which looks at the surfaces of cells. Based on their physical appearance, Dr. Simpson classified the RBCs into six groups, ranging from normal to severely mal-

49

formed.

The CFS patients had many more deformed RBCs than healthy people, Dr. Simpson discovered.

The large percentage of deformed RBCs in people with CFS could result in a reduced ability of these cells to enter small blood vessels, reducing oxygen in those areas, Dr. Simpson concluded.

Although this deformity of the RBCs might contribute to the disease, Dr. Simpson suggested that the discovery might possibly be most helpful as a diagnostic test.

28 People With CFS Develop New Allergies

One reason that people with CFS develop new allergies may be because they produce too much of a chemical called histamine, which controls some types of allergy attacks.

CFS patients—like AIDS patients—become allergic to foods, medications, chemicals (such as hair spray), perfume, and a variety of substances they weren't allergic to before they got sick.

In fact, Dr. Nancy Klimas (at the University of Miami) has found that 70 percent of CFS patients develop new allergies. And Manhattan's Dr. Ronald Hoffman believes that these new allergies are due to an underlying viral infection.

These new allergies are very bothersome to CFS patients, and they almost always describe them when they are discussing their illness.

"David" has developed allergies to "everything" over the last ten years he has been sick: food, chemicals, and medications. Allergy tests revealed allergies to "hundreds of things," David says. But when he tried to be desensitized by an allergist (a typical therapy for multiple allergies), he got much sicker.

CFS patient "Susan" also developed allergies after she became ill. Strangely, Susan's horse developed allergies about the same time as she did. The horse became allergic to the soap he had always been bathed with, to penicillin and other medications, and to the routine immunizations horses receive.

"Friends thought it was funny, the horse developing allergies, because I had food allergies," Susan told me. She had never had allergies before she got CFS. "In fact, I used to be one of those people who thought people with allergies were making too big a deal of them."

This epidemic could be devastating to the perfume industry. One of the "nightmare" situations that CFS patients describe is walking into the perfume section of a store and being overwhelmed by all the different scents.

For a CFS patient, a perfume called Poison can be exactly what the name implies.

29 Histamine May Play A Major Role In CFS

Histamine is a chemical naturally produced in the human body; one of its main functions is to mediate allergic responses. Histamine also governs the release of gastric, or stomach, acids.

Because of histamine's influence on the production of stomach acids, two anti-ulcer medicines have been created to block histamine's action. One is called Tagamet (produced by SmithKline Beecham Pharmaceuticals, Philadelphia) and the other, produced in Britain, is called Zantac (Glaxo Pharmaceuticals, London).

An unusual—and unexpected—effect of both these anti-ulcer medications is the stimulation of natural killer (NK) cell activity. As we will discuss in more detail in a later chapter, NK cell activity—important in fighting viral infections and cancers—is very severely decreased in people with CFS.

Dr. Nancy Klimas (University of Miami) explained very clearly the importance of NK cells in a talk she presented at a conference in Charlotte, NC, in late 1990.

"Natural killer cells are your *primitive* immune system—like back in the era of the dinosaurs," Dr. Klimas said. "Before there were people, there were natural killer cells. To this day, sharks have only natural killer cells to deal with infection. Natural killer cells are *always* charged up and going. . . . Natural killer cells attack anything that's not part of you."

NK cell activity is not only decreased in CFS patients, it is also severely lowered in people with AIDS. A Danish research team recently performed an experiment to measure the impact of Zantac on the NK cell activity of a group of HIV-positive men, compared to a group of HIV-positive men who received a placebo (an inert substance). The results were astounding.

Zantac increased the NK cell activity of the treated men significantly, the Danish researchers found.

Why is this? Well, it isn't really clear, but it is known that histamine acts by binding to a type of immune system cell. When that binding takes place, it is thought, "histamine-induced suppressor factor"—a substance believed to suppress the immune system—is released.

That factor may cause the decrease of NK cell activity seen in people with AIDS and CFS.

Dr. Klimas also found, from a study of the NK cell activity in CFS patients, that their NK cell activity was lowest "of all the populations we've studied," including AIDS patients.

Can an overabundance of histamine cause the symptoms—allergies and gastrointestinal problems—as well as the immunosuppression seen in CFS? If those symptoms are controlled by anti-histamine drugs like Zantac and Tagamet, it would be a good hint that histamine may be causing at least some of the symptoms of CFS. And perhaps most importantly for patients, both Tagamet and Zantac are safe drugs already approved by the Food and Drug Administration!

30 People With CFS Often Can't Drink Alcohol

A very striking symptom that helps doctors differentiate CFS from other illnesses, especially depression, is alcohol intolerance. People with CFS often become very sick when they drink alcohol—even those who previously drank alcohol often.

Alcohol intolerance is often used by physicians when trying to diagnose CFS. Manhattan physician Dr. Ronald Hoffman always asks patients he suspects might have CFS, "How do you feel when you drink?"

"Some people who are depressed are driven to drink," Dr. Hoffman said. "And they reply that when they drink, they don't feel so bad. But people with CFS really feel *toxic* when they drink. As much as they might want to drink, they can't."

Charlotte's Dr. Paul Cheney suspects that this alcohol intolerance may be related to the increased sensitivity to medications that people with CFS develop, he said at a research conference in early 1991.

Why do people with CFS become so sensitive to drugs and alcohol? Some researchers hypothesize it's because of an "up-regulation" of the immune system: That some element in the immune system is turned on and can't seem to be turned off. Therefore, substances once tolerated easily now produce an overreaction by the immune system, making CFS patients sicker.

31 Some People With CFS Become Completely Disabled

Sometimes the symptoms experienced by people with CFS—memory loss, fatigue, pain, and stomach problems—become so severe that they can no longer work. Because CFS is still not considered to be a disabling illness, disability benefits are difficult to get—and CFS patients can lose their jobs, their homes, and their spouses.

"Mark," a CFS patient in California, was the top salesperson at a California cable television company at the age of 23. In fact, he told me, he'd held "every sales record" in the company. But in August 1981, he woke up one day not feeling well, with a sore throat and flu-like symptoms. Mark hasn't been well since.

Mark began "wasting away," lost 20 pounds—and his job. So, like many CFS patients with the option, he moved back home with his parents.

In 1983, Mark decided to try working as a stockbroker, because of the flexible hours. But his memory, which had deteriorated from the time he first became ill, made it almost impossible for him to function as a stockbroker and, in time, he had to quit that job, too.

I recently interviewed a Long Island physician disabled by CFS. He had worked as a doctor for 26 years and had never missed a day's work due to illness. But, two years after his wife developed CFS, the doctor came down with the illness, too. Eight people in his extended household now have symptoms reminiscent of CFS.

Not everyone with CFS becomes completely unable to work. But if even one percent of CFS patients are disabled, the economic costs to the U.S. will soon become staggering.

32 A Very Important Defense Against Viruses And Cancer Doesn't Work In People With CFS

A type of immune system cell called the natural killer (NK) cell doesn't work in people with CFS. NK cells are one of the most important defenses against both viral infections and cancers.

Unlike other immune system cells, which have to be activated by a chemical signal, NK cells attack anything that's not part of the body. That includes not only viruses, but also cancer cells.

Dr. Ronald Herberman (who is a professor at the Cancer Institute at the University of Pittsburgh) has studied NK cell activity in people with CFS. He has also studied the development of cancer in CFS patients—and their close companions—and believes that lowered NK cell activity may allow cancer to develop at a very high rate in CFS patients.

Dr. Herberman studied an outbreak of "epidemic CFS" in a symphony orchestra. When he studied the NK cell activity of the CFS patients in the orchestra, he found that it was abnormally low; in fact, it was about half of what it is in healthy people. He found that some of the "healthy" individuals in the symphony orchestra also had very low NK cell activity.

In her studies, Dr. Nancy Klimas (at the University of Miami) has found that NK cell activity in CFS is patients is as low as she has ever seen for any disease. According to Dr. Klimas, NK cell activity is lower in CFS patients than in patients with AIDS-related complex. Dr. Klimas has concluded that NK cells are very important in CFS.

In her very detailed study of the immune systems of people with CFS, Dr. Klimas found that CFS patients had an NK cell activity deficit of 83 percent.

33 CFS Patients May Develop Cancers More Often Than The General Public

Cancer cells grow in perfectly healthy people from time to time. Not everyone gets cancer, because a healthy immune system identifies cancer cells and kills them before they grow out of control to form tumors.

But in people whose immune systems don't work properly—people who have AIDS or some other immune system disease, or whose immune system has been suppressed chemically because they have received an organ transplant—the abnormal cancer cells *do* grow out of control.

In an outbreak of CFS in a symphony orchestra in 1984, eight of the 58 orchestra members developed typical symptoms of CFS. Dr. Ronald Herberman at the University of Pittsburgh Cancer Institute and other scientists studied the orchestra members—those who didn't get sick, as well as those who did—to get a better understanding of what they called "epidemic CFS."

The team of scientists measured a type of blood cell which is the body's primary defense against both cancer and viruses; this cell is called the "natural killer cell" because its natural function is to kill any cell that is abnormal.

Natural killer cells didn't work properly in the CFS patients in the orchestra, these scientists discovered. But they also didn't work well in some of the "healthy" members of the orchestra. They wondered: Were *all* of the orchestra members infected with a virus that attacks the immune system, but doesn't produce symptoms in some people?

The orchestra members were studied for several years, and during that period, four cancers developed in this young, previously healthy group.

One cancer was a very rare type of blood cell cancer called a B-cell lymphoma. Another orchestra member developed breast cancer; the third had a salivary gland cancer. The fourth cancer was a brain tumor.

These orchestra members were developing cancer at a rate almost 18 percent higher than the general population.

Most alarming of all, half of the cancers developed in people with no symptoms of CFS. Were their immune systems attacked by an "invisible" invader?

It is increasingly recognized by CFS researchers that people with CFS, and their close contacts, develop cancers at a much higher (but not yet determined) rate than people in the general population. Dr. Paul Cheney has found brain cancers to be very common among family members of people with CFS.

In August 1990, the *New York Times* announced an alarming rise in the number of brain cancers occurring world-wide. In the last ten years, the *New York Times* reported, brain cancers had increased by 300 percent across all age groups. The cancer experts who were consulted concluded that the rise was genuine, and not simply the result of better diagnostic tests becoming available.

This world-wide rise in brain cancer may be due to people becoming infected with a virus that suppresses the immune system—causing the symptoms of CFS in some people, and cancer in others.

34 Yeast Infections Can Be Severe

We live peacefully with many types of organisms inside our bodies: viruses, bacteria, and yeast. Some of these organisms perform important duties for our bodies, like helping us to digest food. But when the immune system doesn't limit the number of these organisms to a helpful level, they can grow dangerously out of control and cause disease.

One of the organisms which can become a problem when the immune system is damaged is a type of yeast named Candida; it lives in people's digestive and reproductive systems.

Candida yeast can grow out of control in the mouth and throat, and cause an infection called "thrush." Thrush looks like a white coating of the tongue and mouth, and it is a very common infection in both AIDS and CFS patients.

Female AIDS and CFS patients can develop vaginal yeast infections which are difficult to cure.

These types of yeast infections are a very important warning sign that the immune system is not functioning as it should.

35 CFS Has Been Called An "Acquired Immunodeficiency"

AIDS is an acronym for "Acquired Immune Deficiency Syndrome," so it is especially noteworthy that a June 1990 scientific research report concluded that CFS is "a form of acquired immunodeficiency."

"Immunodeficiency," of course, means that the immune system is unable to perform its usual functions. "Acquired" means that it is caused by outside factors, which could include foreign organisms (viruses, bacteria) or toxic substances (chemical or nuclear waste, for example). Studies of people with CFS have not found any toxic substances to which most patients have been exposed, so researchers now believe that an organism, probably a virus, is attacking the immune systems of CFS patients.

Dr. Nancy Klimas at the University of Miami and her colleagues performed very detailed studies on the immune systems of CFS patients which led them to conclude that the illness is a form of immunodeficiency.

One of the most interesting things that Dr. Klimas and her coworkers discovered was that 70 percent of the CFS patients in their study had developed allergies after becoming sick. Allergies are one type of abnormal immune response.

Dr. Klimas and her colleagues also discovered that some CFS patients produce extremely elevated levels of an immune system-stimulating chemical called interleukin-1. These CFS patients, Dr. Klimas found, can have *50 times* as much interleukin-1 as healthy people.

But probably most importantly, Dr. Klimas's group discovered that the natural killer cells, blood cells which kill foreign invaders as well as cancer cells, didn't work well at all in CFS patients. The natural killer cells in this group of CFS patients showed a decreased killing ability of 83 percent. This dramatic decrease was similar to that seen in intravenous drug users, Dr. Klimas and her colleagues pointed out.

Dr. Klimas found that evidence of immune deficiency was present in all of the CFS patients studied by her research group.

36 CFS Shares Many Disturbing Characteristics With AIDS

Both AIDS and CFS are conditions in which the immune system breaks down. But they have other features in common as well.

Both are "syndromes," or collections of symptoms varying in number and intensity among patients. AIDS and CFS share quite a number of symptoms, especially in the beginning: fever, fatigue, night sweats, lymph node pain, nervous system abnormalities, and gastrointestinal problems.

Both sets of patients can develop a yeast infection of the mouth and throat called "thrush." AIDS and CFS patients develop allergies, especially to medications.

AIDS and CFS patients develop the same types of nervous system problems: difficulty in remembering, confusion, dizziness, mood swings, weakness, impaired coordination, difficulty in reading and writing, depression, and eye diseases.

And researchers are increasingly finding that CFS patients—like AIDS patients—develop cancers at a much higher rate than the general population.

That may be because, as studies are now showing, a type of blood cell called natural killer (NK) cell does not work properly in people with AIDS or CFS. Natural killer cells are one of the first, and most important, defenses the immune system mounts against foreign invaders and cancer cells.

People with CFS or AIDS also have very high antibodies against some of the same viruses: cytomegalovirus (which can cause blindness), Epstein-Barr Virus (which was suspected to cause both syndromes when they were first discovered), and a newly discovered virus called Human Herpes Virus 6 (HHV-6).

HHV-6 has been shown to infect and kill both immune system and nervous system cells. It is such an efficient killer of immune system cells that it has been suggested as a possible cause or "cofactor" in the development of AIDS. HHV-6 is also currently being investigated as a possible cause of CFS.

An unknown percentage of AIDS patients is infected with a newly discovered type of bacterium called a mycoplasma. This bacterium not only attacks the immune system and eludes its surveillance, it also causes organ tissues (like kidneys) to rot. There is some evidence that CFS patients may be infected with this mycoplasma but, as with AIDS, there is no hard evidence of how many CFS patients may harbor the organism.

Will AIDS and CFS be found to be different forms of the same illness, caused when a virus (like HHV-6) or bacteria (like the mycoplasma) attacks the immune system?

We don't know the answer to that question yet. We do know, however, that the immune systems in AIDS and CFS patients are damaged in strikingly similar ways and that they develop many similar types of problems, including nervous system diseases, infections, and cancer. For some, the connection between the two syndromes is too frightening to contemplate.

37 A Swine Illness Is Very Similar To CFS. CFS May Be Caused By African Swine Fever Virus

There is an illness of swine, called African Swine Fever, that can produce a chronic illness that is quite similar to CFS. It can also produce an extremely acute form of illness that pigs' immune systems are unable to fight; and it can kill them very quickly. Understanding this illness of pigs could lead to a greater understanding of why so many organ systems are affected by CFS and why the symptoms are more severe in some people than in others—it could explain the relationship, if there is one, between CFS and AIDS. Some scientists think it is the cause of both syndromes.

Does it seem odd to look at a swine illness to try to explain a human disease? It isn't, really; the human and porcine (swine) immune systems are very similar. Pigs are a major repository for human influenza viruses, and passage from humans to pigs and back to humans accounts in part for the wide variety of strains of influenza from year to year.

African Swine Fever is caused by a virus, African Swine Fever Virus (ASFV). Before the turn of the century, ASFV existed as a non-disease-producing infection in African warthogs; around 1900, however, the virus jumped species and somehow became capable of infecting domestic swine.

Many different strains of ASFV exist at any one time, causing five forms of African Swine Fever in pigs: hyperacute, acute, subacute, chronic, and subclinical or inapparent (in which "carrier pigs" are not sick themselves but can infect others).

In hyperacute ASF, pigs usually die one to three days after they first appear to be sick, and 100 percent of a herd can die. The symptoms are high fever, accelerated breathing, patches of skin engorged with blood; sick pigs stop eating and lose weight. The nervous system is also affected by ASFV; infected pigs have trouble standing and moving, and are not alert. Sometimes they have seizures.

The symptoms of ASF are somewhat less life-threatening in the acute and subacute forms, although miscarriages can occur. Fewer

60

pigs die (60-90 percent, instead of 100), and they live longer (six to ten days).

Pigs who survive the sub-acute form of ASF develop chronic disease. They have recurring fevers and lack of alertness; they lose their appetites and weight, or fail to grow. Skin lesions and arthritis can develop, and pneumonia is very common. The symptoms usually last several months, waxing and waning in severity.

Pigs often recover from chronic ASF, but they can die from pneumonia, heart failure, or becoming re-infected with a more deadly strain of the virus.

The ASF virus is a remarkable invader of the immune system: It is capable of destroying immune system cells, and the immune system cannot make antibodies that destroy it. The virus can infect the spleen, lymph nodes, lung, liver, kidney, tonsils, and brain.

The virus is also constantly changing; this has impeded efforts to create a vaccine against it. And even when scientists have been able to create a vaccine against one strain of ASFV, the vaccinated animal is still vulnerable to infection by other strains of the virus.

Studying ASFV proves that one virus can cause relapsing symptoms affecting many different systems in the body, and is a good model for what happens in CFS. If CFS is caused by an as-yet-unidentified virus, that virus may act very similarly to ASFV.

38 U.S. Government Health Authorities Have Done Little To Investigate CFS

Ask just about any question about CFS, and the answer most likely will be: "Nothing has been proven conclusively." Even the National Institute of Allergy and Infectious Diseases, the U.S. government agency primarily responsible for studying CFS, referred to the "dearth of scientifically sound information" about CFS in a summary of its own research for 1991.

As of December 1990, only five research projects to study CFS had been funded by the National Institute of Allergy and Infectious Diseases. Only about two-and-a-half million dollars was spent by that agency to study CFS in 1991.

The Centers for Disease Control in Atlanta, the government agency in charge of tracking epidemics of old and new diseases, spent only about $2 million in 1991 to determine how many Americans may already have CFS.

That comes to a grand total of $4.5 million spent in 1991 by U.S. health agencies to investigate an epidemic that some experts estimate may already affect as many as 10 million Americans.

In July 1991, a CFS patient organization called CACTUS (which stands for CFIDS Action Campaign for the United States) compared the amount of federal research money spent to study various immune system illnesses.

CACTUS found that, for every AIDS patient, the U.S. government spends $750 in research money. For every patient with the autoimmune disorder lupus, $79 is spent; for every patient with multiple sclerosis, another immune system disorder, $28 is spent.

One dollar and thirty-three cents ($1.33) is spent in federal research dollars for each estimated CFS patient in the U.S.

39 The CDC Surveillance Study Is Slow Going

In 1986, the Congressional Subcommittee on Appropriations —the Subcommittee that gives government agencies money to run on and guides how that money is spent—instructed the Centers for Disease Control (CDC) to establish a "reporting protocol" for CFS by the end of 1987. A reporting protocol instructs physicians how to report a disease to the CDC so that the number of people with the illness can be measured.

As of December 1991, the reporting protocol that Congress had requested five years prior still did not exist.

It is still unknown how many Americans may have CFS. Private sector researchers, however, estimate that as many as 3-10 million people may already have CFS in the U.S.

If even the smaller estimate—three million—is correct, twice as many Americans already have CFS as are thought to be infected with HIV, the virus believed by many researchers to cause AIDS.

The nation is in a panic over the AIDS epidemic; yet many people are unaware that another illness of immune deficiency, CFS, may be much more widespread than AIDS.

What has the CDC, charged with safeguarding the American public against outbreaks of epidemic illnesses, been doing about CFS?

The CDC did, in late 1988, begin what is called a "surveillance study" to estimate how widespread CFS is. Published results from that study will not be available until mid-1992.

Four sites were selected for the surveillance study: Atlanta, Reno, Grand Rapids, and Wichita. CFS, like AIDS, appears to have "hot spots" in major cities like New York City, Miami, San Francisco, and Los Angeles; however, the surveillance study is not surveying any of those cities.

The CDC's Dr. Walter Gunn presented preliminary findings from the surveillance study at a CFS conference in November 1990 (held in Charlotte, NC). Dr. Gunn discussed findings from 147 of the 284 people who had agreed to participate in the CDC's study.

Dr. Gunn announced at this conference that 26-27 percent of the 147 patients fully met the CDC criteria for CFS. Another 18 percent came within a symptom or two of fully meeting the criteria. He said that these findings were very surprising to the research team at CDC, because they had expected that only 3-5 percent of the patients studied would fully meet the CDC criteria—yet 26-27 percent met that definition! Another 18 percent almost met the definition, bringing the grand total to 44-45 percent—almost half!

So ten times as many people as the CDC expected may meet the agency's own definition for the illness. As patients and patient advocates have long argued, the CDC and other government health agencies have seriously underestimated how widespread the CFS epidemic already has become in the United States.

In October 1991, Dr. Gunn told the *Atlanta Constitution* that the name of the syndrome should be changed, perhaps to "Chronic

Immune Deficiency Syndrome." Such a name would suggest that CFS is a lot more like AIDS than many people would like to admit.

40 Scientists Outside The U.S. Take CFS Very Seriously

Unlike the American medical establishment, led by federal health institutes with little interest in CFS, researchers around the world take CFS very seriously indeed.

For instance, researchers in Australia recently studied an area of the continent which has a population of 114,000. They estimate that approximately one out of every 3,000 people in Australia has CFS.

In Japan, CFS was named "Low Natural Killer Syndrome" because natural killer cells do not work properly in people with CFS. Japanese researchers did not stop with defining the illness, however; they experimented with a drug developed from extracts of shiitake mushroom, long believed in Japan to have immune-stimulating properties. The Japanese researchers found that after six months of treatment with the drug (named lentinan), the CFS patients appeared to be almost completely recovered.

In Canada, researchers at the University of Alberta (Edmonton) and Dalhousie University (Halifax) are studying the effect of CFS on the heart. Preliminary studies have shown that CFS patients experience a slow increase in heart rates, causing them to tire more easily and more quickly than healthy people. And a Toronto physician who has seen more than 1,000 CFS patients, Dr. Anne Mildon, has told reporters that some of her CFS patients are losing their sight; others are too weak to move.

Researchers in other countries—including England, Scotland, Germany, and New Zealand—are studying various aspects of CFS while much of the U.S. medical establishment is still debating whether the disease exists.

41 No One Knows What Causes CFS (Or No One Admits They Know What Causes It)

CFS is often described as a "mystery illness" because no one knows what causes it. The lack of a proven cause also has contributed to skepticism about it being a "real" illness in the press and the medical establishment, and to early theories of it being a psychological illness.

Some of these theories about CFS suggested that it might be caused by an environmental toxin; tung oil, heavy metals such as mercury—even the amalgam that is used in filling tooth cavities—have been suspected. None of these substances has ever been convincingly tied to CFS.

Research during the last few years has uncovered very specific perturbations in the immune systems and nervous systems of people with CFS. These newly-described physiological abnormalities, as well as the tendency for CFS to occur in "clusters" or groups of people, now have convinced most CFS researchers that the syndrome is caused by an infectious agent.

Another early theory suggested that CFS was caused by the Epstein-Barr Virus (EBV), because some patients had very high levels of antibodies to this virus. In fact, one of the first names given to the syndrome was "Chronic Epstein-Barr Virus," or CEBV, Syndrome. Because EBV causes mononucleosis, CFS has also been called "chronic mononucleosis syndrome."

But because about 99 percent of the world's population has antibodies to EBV that rise and fall in number depending on the health of the immune system, EBV is now recognized as a type of early warning system. When antibodies to EBV rise in an individual, it usually means that something else is attacking the immune system.

Numerous groups of researchers around the world are now working feverishly to be the first to identify the infectious agent that causes CFS.

But given the rather clear and convincing data emerging from current research that a virus that also infects AIDS patients, Human Herpes Virus-6 or HHV-6, is the real culprit, it is hard to believe that top government scientists don't know what is going on.

42 People With CFS Are Infected With A Virus That Infects AIDS Patients

The AIDS epidemic has resulted in an explosion in the field of virology, the study of viruses. As a result of new techniques and increasing expertise, a number of new human (and animal) viruses have been discovered in the last ten years.

One of those viruses, first isolated from AIDS and cancer patients, is called Human Herpes Virus Type 6, or HHV-6.

Although it has recently been suggested that much of the world population is infected with HHV-6, it appears to make some people very, very sick. Some researchers have suggested that there are different types, or strains, of HHV-6 and that some are more harmful than others.

In the laboratory, HHV-6 causes many types of cells—especially immune system and nervous system cells—to clump together in balloon-like structures and then die.

HHV-6 is such an effective killer of immune system cells that some scientists have suggested that it is a "co-factor," or helper, in the development of AIDS.

Patients with CFS also have very high levels of antibodies to HHV-6, and some researchers have suggested that their immune systems are being attacked by this virus.

HHV-6 has been associated with fatal hepatitis (liver disease), and also has been found in brain tissue, as well as in several types of cancer tissue. Some studies have suggested that HHV-6 can cause some kinds of cancers.

HHV-6 is found in saliva, and it probably passes from person to person through exchanges of saliva: coughing, kissing, and sharing food utensils.

One newspaper which has covered the CFS epidemic extensively, the *New York Native*, has argued that HHV-6 is really not a herpes virus, but is actually African Swine Fever Virus, the same virus that causes chronic immune dysfunction in pigs.

Currently, there is an epidemic of an illness in pigs all over the world called Swine Mystery Disease. Pigs with the disease show signs of immune dysfunction.

The *New York Native* has suggested that pigs may be infected with the same virus that is found in AIDS and CFS patients, HHV-6—which the *Native* argues has been mis-identified, and which is actually African Swine Fever Virus.

43 A Virus Similar To The AIDS Virus Has Been Found In People With CFS

AIDS is generally believed to be caused by the Human Immunodeficiency Virus, HIV (although a growing number of scientists are questioning that belief, since it has never been shown *how* HIV causes any of the illnesses seen in AIDS patients). HIV is a retrovirus; instead of being made up of DNA (the cell's genetic material), like most disease-causing viruses, it is made up of RNA, a related compound.

Two groups of scientists have discovered what they believe to be new retroviruses in CFS patients. This work is very preliminary, and new information is being made public nearly every week. So far, it is not even known whether the two groups of scientists are working with the same retrovirus.

This work is also very controversial; some scientists doubt that what has been discovered in CFS patients' blood is a retrovirus at all.

If a new retrovirus—or more than one—has been found in CFS patients, it is not necessarily the cause of the syndrome. The retrovirus(es) may turn out to be harmless, or only harmful to people whose immune systems have already been attacked and weakened by some other infectious agent.

The discovery of retroviruses in CFS patients, whatever its role, strengthens the argument that CFS and AIDS are part of a family of immune system illnesses.

44 Some Information About CFS Has Been Concealed By U.S. Health Officials

Many CFS patients are distrustful of U.S. health officials—at the Centers for Disease Control (CDC) and the National Institutes of Health (NIH)—because those agencies have been so slow to do anything about the illness. In some instances, the health agencies supposed to be protecting the public health have concealed important information about CFS from the public.

Using the Freedom of Information Act, I have uncovered documents that prove that certain government health officials have intentionally misled the public.

For instance, when the CDC investigated the first recognized outbreak of CFS in 1986, the investigator in charge *altered the data from the outbreak when he published his findings in a scientific journal.* The data were so blatantly falsified that Dr. Paul Cheney, one of the physicians who recognized the outbreak, refused to attach his name to the scientific report published by the CDC official.

The same CDC official was informed in mid-1988 that CFS patients appeared to be developing cancers at a rate much higher than expected. Instead of investigating further, this official simply stated that CFS patients who developed cancer were no longer CFS patients—they were cancer patients.

Former Surgeon General C. Everett Koop was informed in spring 1987 that CFS was occurring in outbreaks all over the country among health care workers. Dr. Koop has never publicly discussed CFS—while Surgeon General or since leaving office—or tried to warn the nation that it is a contagious illness.

Officials at the NIH also have possessed information for several years about the contagious nature of CFS as well as the possibility that cancer is very common in not only CFS patients but also their "healthy" family members and co-workers. But NIH scientists have been silent about this contagious illness which some CFS researchers now estimate may already affect ten million Americans; in fact, the leading CFS researcher at NIH, Dr. Stephen Straus, continues to assert that CFS is a psychological illness.

Why are U.S. health officials engaged in a cover-up of the true facts about CFS? (There are only *two* federal research projects studying CFS, one at NIH and one at CDC, so it doesn't require much collusion to create a cover-up of the facts.)

A physician told me that NIH's head CFS researcher, when pressed to explain why he continues to describe CFS as a psychological illness, admitted: "We don't want a public panic."

45 Most Insurance Companies Won't Pay For Tests Or Treatments

There is no treatment for CFS approved by the Food and Drug Administration (FDA), although a number of drugs are being tested on CFS patients. There is no specific diagnostic test for CFS, even though certain laboratory tests can pretty well confirm whether a person has CFS.

Because of these two facts—there is no FDA-approved treatment and no diagnostic test—most insurance companies refuse to pay for either treatments or laboratory tests for CFS. They are considered "experimental." And insurance companies are not required to pay for experimental treatments or tests.

But many of the tests performed on CFS patients to determine the level of functioning of their immune and nervous systems—blood tests, brain scans, tests to measure intellectual capacity—work in a well-established and accepted manner.

And they can be very expensive.

Insurance companies must be convinced that CFS is a very real, and very debilitating, illness; otherwise, they will continue refusing to pay for tests and treatments.

Given the fact that the whole population is at risk for developing the syndrome, this epidemic could devastate the insurance industry.

If and when there is a test for CFS, insurance companies can be expected to use it to screen applicants who try to obtain health insurance, a sobering prospect.

46 Disability Benefits Are Difficult For CFS Patients To Get

Many CFS patients are living in tragic situations: Marriages dissolve, jobs are lost, and many CFS patients are abandoned by their families because they aren't believed to have a "real" disease. As a result, many CFS patients are flat broke, lose their homes or apartments, and become very isolated—on top of being very sick.

Both private and public disability insurance is extremely difficult for CFS patients to get because the illness is not treated seriously either by government health agencies or the medical profession in general.

I recently interviewed a physician who developed CFS after 26 years of practicing medicine. He had faithfully paid for disability insurance for those 26 years; yet, when he was no longer able to work because of CFS, his insurance company at first refused to pay him disability benefits.

Being a doctor, this CFS patient eventually convinced his insurer that he was truly ill and unable to work. But if even a physician with the illness has to fight to obtain the disability benefits he has paid for for 26 years, what is a younger person with less clout supposed to do?

Even if one million people are disabled by CFS—and remember, some experts suggest that three to ten million Americans may already have the illness—it will have a devastating effect on the economy.

Both public (Social Security Administration) and private disability insurers could be bankrupted by a catastrophe like ten million Americans becoming disabled.

Which makes it all the more urgent for CFS to be investigated with the full power of U.S. health agencies behind such research.

47 A New Drug May Help People With CFS

A fairly new drug, called Ampligen, has shown some promise in treating both CFS and AIDS patients. Ampligen has not been approved by the Food and Drug Administration (FDA) for treatment of either syndrome, but clinical trials are being conducted that some researchers think will show that Ampligen is safe and effective.

In a very small clinical trial of 15 CFS patients in 1989, Ampligen appeared to improve patients' IQ, memory, and exercise tolerance.

This small Ampligen study also produced more evidence that Human Herpes Virus Type 6 (HHV-6) may be responsible for causing some of the symptoms of CFS. In patients who improved while on Ampligen, levels of antibodies to HHV-6 decreased dramatically. Those patients who were not helped by Ampligen demonstrated no decrease in HHV-6 antibody levels.

What is Ampligen and how does it work?

Ampligen is a type of RNA molecule. RNA is a relative of DNA, which contains the genetic code; some types of RNA help DNA genes reproduce. RNA also is the substance that retroviruses are composed of (unlike conventional viruses, which are made up of DNA).

It isn't known exactly how Ampligen works, but some studies have suggested that the drug corrects a defect in an important immune pathway disturbed by viral infections. Ampligen is thought to stimulate the immune system and to possess anti-viral properties.

Ampligen also is capable of crossing the blood-brain barrier, the very important defense system that protects the brain from harmful chemicals and infectious agents. Unfortunately, the blood-brain barrier is so efficient that it can also block beneficial, disease-fighting agents from entering the brain. Ampligen appears to be able to circumvent that protective barrier.

The only documented side effects from Ampligen treatment so

71

far are mild flu-like symptoms; none of the 15 patients in the 1990 study stopped Ampligen therapy because of those apparently minor side effects.

48 The Japanese May Already Have Discovered An Effective Treatment For CFS

Since 1969, Japanese researchers have been studying a compound extracted from shiitake mushrooms: It is called lentinan. Lentinan was studied first as a cancer treatment; more recently, it has been studied as a treatment for immune system disorders like CFS and AIDS.

Lentinan is thought to have virus-fighting and immune-stimulating properties; it is thought to work by stimulating production of the anti-cancer and anti-virus substance interferon.

Lentinan also has been shown to stimulate the activity of natural killer (NK) cells, which are the body's first line of defense against both viruses and tumors.

In 1987, Japanese researchers defined a new illness which they called "Low Natural Killer Syndome" (LNKS). The symptoms of LNKS are strikingly similar to CFS, and the two illnesses appear to be identical.

These Japanese researchers treated a group of 23 LNKS patients with lentinan (which must be administered intravenously). After only 2-4 weeks of treatment, the patients regained a sense of well-being.

After six months of lentinan therapy, the patients' natural killer cell activity was restored to normal levels.

Because lentinan is delivered by injection, it is classified as a drug by the U.S. Food and Drug Administration.

Another shiitake mushroom extract, used as a food supplement in Japan for more than ten years and taken orally, recently has become available over-the-counter in the United States. It is named LEM.

LEM, like lentinan, appears to have tumor-inhibiting and immune-stimulating properties. LEM has been shown to protect liver cells (in the laboratory) from toxic chemicals, and appears to be beneficial in treating chronic liver disease.

After more than 20 years of study (mostly conducted in Japan), neither lentinan nor LEM has been shown to produce any deleterious side effects.

49 You Can Help Speed Up Research By Writing To Congress

CFS is rapidly becoming *everyone*'s problem. If, as some experts speculate, as many as ten million Americans already have CFS, it will soon become a major public health problem touching every citizen's life.

Congress is aware that CFS is a growing public health problem, and it has been asking for accelerated research from both the Centers for Disease Control (CDC) and the National Institutes of Health (NIH) for a number of years.

The more constituents a Congressional representative hears from about a particular problem, the more attention he or she will be inclined to devote to it.

If you are concerned about CFS, you can write letters to your federal representatives in Congress.

Local public health officials also have to be made aware that people are increasingly concerned about CFS. In San Francisco, where the CFIDS Foundation has lobbied local health officials relentlessly, CFS has been declared a major health problem.

Local officials *do* respond to requests for information about what is being done to fight public health problems. You can call your city and state health departments and ask them what is being done about CFS. Mayors' and governors' offices usually have health liaisons whose jobs are to respond to inquiries from the public about health-related matters.

Information about what is being done by the CDC and the NIH can be obtained by telephoning or writing to the Public Information Offices of those agencies. They often will supply information about illnesses being investigated free of charge to the public.

50 There Are Chronic Fatigue Syndrome Organizations That Can Help Victims Of CFS

Organizations of CFS patients have been formed all over the country. These organizations provide emotional support and various levels of practical help to CFS patients and their families. Some organizations refer patients to doctors knowledgeable about CFS, and most have a newsletter of some type that disseminates information about research and funding.

The two biggest national organizations (with the most informative newsletters) are located in Charlotte, North Carolina (The CFIDS Association) and in San Francisco (The CFIDS Foundation).

The CFIDS Association publishes a newsletter called the *CFIDS Chronicle*, sent to members who pay a small membership fee. Through the *CFIDS Chronicle*, various types of literature about the illness also are made available. You can write to the CFIDS Association at P.O. Box 220398, Charlotte, NC 28222-0398.

The CFIDS Association, along with an advocacy group called the CFIDS Action Campaign for The United States (CACTUS), have established a toll-free number that uses a voice mail-box system to provide information about CFS at no cost to the caller. That number is: 800-442-3437.

Another phone service established by CACTUS and the CFIDS Association is not free, but provides information on medical and research topics. The cost is $2.00 for the first minute, and $1.00 for each additional minute. That number is: 900-988-2343.

CACTUS is a national coalition of CFS organizations formed

to lobby for increased funding, research, and services for people with CFS from all levels of government, as well as to disseminate information to members. For more information about CACTUS, write to P.O. Box 2578, Sebastopol, CA 95473.

The CFIDS Foundation publishes a newsletter called *CFIDS Treatment News*. The CFIDS Foundation can be reached at 965 Mission Street, Suite 425, San Francisco, CA 94103.

Many cities have formed local CFS support groups; check your local telephone directory to find out if there is a group in your area.

Afterword

In December 1991, two major developments in the evolving Chronic Fatigue Syndrome story occurred—both of which strengthened the hypothesis that there is a connection between CFS and AIDS.

The Associate Director of the Centers for Disease Control Tuberculosis Division, Dr. Donald E. Kopanoff, made some startling statements regarding CFS to *Spin* magazine's Victoria Brownworth. In an interview about the widening tuberculosis epidemic, Dr. Kopanoff suggested that CFS patients are at increased risk for contracting TB—and, perhaps, AIDS.

"Chronic fatigue syndrome is so new a disease in terms of our knowledge of it that we simply have no data on whether CFS predisposes someone to TB or even HIV," Dr. Kopanoff told *Spin*. "What we *do* know, categorically and historically, is that people who are in generally poor health are more susceptible to being infected. Severe CFS would cause such a degree of overall poor health that it would be difficult to ward off infection. Yes, those people [CFS patients] *are* at greater risk."

Dr. Kopanoff is the first government health official who has indicated that CFS patients—like AIDS patients—are vulnerable to other, contagious (and in the case of TB, potentially fatal) illnesses

75

because their immune systems are compromised.

The second major development was the publication of a research report about a study conducted at the National Institute of Allergy and Infectious Diseases. Dr. Stephen E. Straus and colleagues, who continue to attempt to link CFS to depression or other psychiatric conditions, discovered a hormonal imbalance in CFS patients.

The hormone they studied is one that is elevated in people suffering from depression. It is cortisol, which is released by the adrenal glands (which are near the kidneys) in response to stress.

Cortisol deficiency is, perhaps not coincidentally, the most common hormonal defect identified in AIDS patients.

In people with CFS, cortisol levels are very low (the opposite of what is seen in depressed people, but exactly like what is seen in AIDS patients). Dr. Straus and colleagues studied the complex pathway that results in cortisol production, and concluded that, in CFS patients, there is most likely a defective signal from the brain. That is, a portion of the brain sends the signal that results in cortisol production; in CFS patients, that signal is insufficient for proper amounts of cortisol to be released.

A lack of cortisol can cause some of the symptoms CFS patients suffer: fatigue, lethargy, feverishness, joint and muscle pain, increased allergies, and disturbances in mood and sleep.

While the impaired hormonal pathway is unlikely to be the cause of CFS, this defect may give researchers valuable clues about the cause of this debilitating syndrome—and what, if any, relationship it has to the other, new illness of immune deficiency, AIDS.

Selected Articles From The Scientific Literature

Presentations made at a Chronic Fatigue Syndrome conference jointly sponsored by the National Institute of Allergy and Infectious Diseases and the University of Pittsburgh (September 15-16, 1988, in Pittsburgh), "Considerations in the Design of Studies of Chronic Fatigue Syndrome," are collected in *Reviews of Infectious Diseases*, Volume 13, Supplement 1, January-February 1991, University of Chicago Press.

Other selected reports in the medical/scientific literature that provide the scientific basis for statements made in this volume include:

Ablashi, D.V. et al.; "Human B-Lymphotropic Virus (Human Herpesvirus-6)"; *Journal of Virological Methods* 21:29, 1988.

Aoki, Tadao et al.; "Antibodies to HTLV-I and -III in Sera from Two Japanese Patients, One With Possible Pre-AIDS"; *Lancet*, October 20, 1984.

Aoki, Tadao, et al.; "Low Natural Killer Syndrome: Clinical and Immunologic Features"; *Natural Immunity and Cell Growth Regulation* 6:116, 1987.

Asano, Yoshizo et al.; "Fatal Fulminate Hepatitis in an Infant With Human Herpesvirus-6 Infection"; *Lancet*, April 7, 1990.

Barnes, Deborah; "Mystery Disease at Lake Tahoe Challenges Virologists and Clinicians"; *Science* 234:541, 1986.

Becker, Yechiel, Editor; *African Swine Fever*, Martinus Nijhoff Publishing (Boston/Dordrecht/Lancaster), 1987.

Behan, P.O. et al.; "The Postviral Fatigue Syndrome: An Analysis of the Findings in 50 Cases"; *Journal of Infection* 10:211, 1985.

Beldekas, John et al.; "African Swine Fever Virus and AIDS"; *Lancet*, March 8, 1986.

Buchwald, Dedra, John L. Sullivan, and Anthony L. Komaroff; "Frequency of 'Chronic Active Epstein-Barr Virus Infection' in a General Medical Practice"; *Journal of the American Medical Association* 257:2303, 1987.

Carter, W. et al.; "Clinical, Immunological, and Virological Effects of Ampligen, a Mismatched Double-Stranded RNA, in Patients With AIDS or AIDS-Related Complex"; *Lancet* 1987, 1228.

Carter, W.; interview in "Experimental Drug Held Effective for Chronic Fatigue, Immune Dysfunction"; American Society for Microbiology *Conference Journal*, September 29-October 2, 1991.

Cheney, Paul R.; "The Chronic Fatigue and Immune Dysfunction Syndrome as a Rising Menace to Public Health"; Congressional testimony delivered May 1989.

DeFreitas, Elaine et al.; "Retroviral Sequences Related to Human T-Lymphotropic Virus Type II in Patients With Chronic Fatigue Immune Dysfunction Syndrome"; *Proceedings of the National Academy of Sciences USA* 88:2922, 1991.

Demitrack, Mark A., Janet K. Dale, Stephen E. Straus et al.; "Evidence for Impaired Activation of the Hypothalamic-Pituitary-Adrenal Axis in Patients With Chronic Fatigue Syndrome"; *Journal of Clinical Endocrinology and Metabolism*, December 1991.

"Gallo Lab Plans Studies to Determine HHV-6 Cofactor Role in AIDS"; *CDC AIDS Weekly*, September 12, 1988.

Grufferman, S. et al.; "Epidemiologic Investigation of an Outbreak of Chronic Fatigue-Immune Dysfunction Syndrome in a Defined Population"; *American Journal of Epidemiology*, Vol. 128, No. 4, 1988.

Harvey, William T.; "A Flight Surgeon's Personal View of an Emerging Illness"; *Aviation, Space, and Environmental Medicine*, December 1989.

Holmes, Gary P. et al.; "Chronic Fatigue Syndrome: A Working Case Definition"; *Annals of Internal Medicine* 108:387, 1988.

Josephs, S.F. et al.; "Genomic Analysis of the Human B-Lymphotropic Virus (HBLV)"; *Science* 234:601, 1986.

Josephs, S.F. et al.; "HHV-6 Reactivation in Chronic Fatigue Syndrome"; *Lancet* 337:1346, June 1, 1991.

Klimas, Nancy G. et al.; "Immunologic Abnormalities in Chronic Fatigue Syndrome"; *Journal of Clinical Microbiology*, June 1990.

Komaroff, A. et al.; "A Chronic 'Post-Viral' Fatigue Syndrome

With Neurologic Features: Serologic Association With Human Herpes Virus-6"; *Abstracts from the Society of General Internal Medicine*, April 27-29, 1988.

Levy, Jay A. et al.; "Frequent Isolation of HHV-6 From Saliva and High Seroprevalence of the Virus in the Population"; *Lancet*, May 5, 1990.

Lo, Shyh-Ching et al.; "Association of the Virus-Like Infectious Agent Originally Reported in Patients With AIDS With Acute Fatal Disease in Previously Healthy Non-AIDS Patients"; *Journal of Tropical Medicine and Hygiene* 41:364, 1989.

Lusso, P. et al.; "Diverse Tropism of Human B-Lymphotropic Virus (Human Herpesvirus 6)"; *Lancet*, September 27, 1987.

Lusso, P. et al.; "In Vitro Cellular Tropism of Human B-Lymphotropic Virus (Human Herpesvirus-6)"; *Journal of Experimental Medicine* 167:1659, May 1988.

Lusso, P. et al.; "In Vitro Susceptibility of T Lymphocytes From Chimpanzees (*Pan troglodytes*) to Human Herpesvirus 6 (HHV-6): A Potential Animal Model to Study the Interaction Between HHV-6 and Human Immunodeficiency Virus Type 1 In Vivo"; *Journal of Virology* 64(6):2751, June 1990.

Lusso, P. et al.; "Induction of CD4 and Susceptibility to HIV-1 Infection in Human CD8 + T Lymphocytes by Human Herpesvirus 6"; *Nature* 349:533, February 7, 1991.

Macek, Catherine; "Acquired Immunodeficiency Syndrome Cause(s) Still Elusive"; *Journal of the American Medical Association* 248:1423, 1982.

Maeda, Yukiko and Goro Chihara; "Lentinan, a New Immuno-accelerator of Cell-Mediated Responses"; *Nature*, February 26, 1971.

Mukherjee, T. et al.; "Abnormal Red Blood Cell Morphology in Myalgic Encephalomyelitis"; *Lancet*, 1987, ii:328.

Murdoch, J. Campbell; "Myalgic Encephalomyelitis (ME) Syndrome—An Analysis of the Clinical Findings in 200 Cases"; *New Zealand Family Physician* 14:51, Autumn 1987.

Murdoch, J. Campbell; "Cell Mediated Immunity in Patients With Myalgic Encephalomyelitis Syndrome"; *New Zealand Medical Journal*, August 10, 1988, 511.

Nanba, Hiroaki and Hisatora Kuroda; "Antitumor Mechanisms of Orally Administered Shiitake Fruit Bodies"; *Chem. Pharm. Bull.* 35:2453, 1987.

Regush, Nicholas; "Health Officials to Issue Alert on Fatigue Syndrome"; *Montreal Gazette*, February 18, 1990.

Salahuddin, S. Zaki et al.; "Isolation of a New Virus, HBLV, in Patients With Lymphoproliferative Disorders"; *Science* 234:596, 1986.

Straus, Stephen E.; "The Chronic Mononucleosis Syndrome"; *Journal of Infectious Diseases*, 1988, 157:405.

Straus, Stephen E. et al.; "Allergy and the Chronic Fatigue Syndrome"; *Journal of Allergy and Clinical Immunology* 81:791, May 1988.

Straus, Stephen E. et al.; "Acyclovir Treatment of the Chronic Fatigue Syndrome"; *New England Journal of Medicine*, December 29, 1988, 1692.

Streicher, H.Z. et al.; "Human Herpes Virus-6 (Human Lymphotropic Virus) Serology in Patients With the Chronic Fatigue Syndrome"; abstract submitted to the Forty-fifth Annual National Meeting of the American Federation for Clinical Research in Washington, DC, April 29-May 2, 1988.

Taijiri, H. et al.; "Human Herpesvirus-6 Infection With Liver Injury in Neonatal Hepatitis"; *Lancet*, April 7, 1990.

Teas, Jane; "Could AIDS Agent Be A New Variant of African Swine Fever Virus?"; *Lancet*, April 23, 1983.

Tochikura, T.S. et al.; "Inhibition (in vitro) of Replication and of the Cytopathic Effect of Human Immunodeficiency Virus by an Extract of the Culture Medium of *Lentinus edodes* Mycelia"; *Medical Microbiology and Immunology* 177:235 (1988), Springer-Verlag International.

A more complete bibliography of scientific articles about Chronic Fatigue Syndrome can be found in *What Really Killed Gilda Radner? Frontline Reports on the Chronic Fatigue Syndrome Epidemic*, by Neenyah Ostrom, copyright © 1991 TNM, Inc.

Index

EBV *see Epstein-Barr Virus;*
see also Chronic Epstein-
Barr Virus (CEBV)
endometriosis 35
epidemic 17, 20, 23, 24, 26,
9, 31, 45, 46, 51, 54, 55,
62, 63, 66, 69
Epstein-Barr Virus (EBV) 65;
see also Chronic Epstein-
Barr Virus (CEBV)
exercise intolerance 30, 33, 34
eye disease 38

fatigue 17, 19, 20, 27, 30, 31,
34, 36, 38, 41, 53, 58, 76
FDA *see Food and Drug Ad-*
ministration
fever 17, 23, 25, 30, 31, 48,
58, 60, 76
fingerprints 48, 49
flu 17, 19, 28, 30, 37, 53, 72
Food and Drug Administra-
tion (FDA) 52, 69, 71, 72

Gunn, Walter 20, 63

Handleman, Marshall J. 42,
43
headaches 17, 18, 27, 30, 48
heart problems 34, 36, 61, 64
Herberman, Ronald 24, 54,
55
HHV-6 *see Human Herpes*
Virus-6
histamines 37, 50, 51, 52
HIV *see Human Immunodefi-*
ciency Virus
Hoffman, Ronald 21, 33, 50,
53
hormones 35, 75

Human Herpes Virus-6
(HHV-6) 27, 48, 59, 65,
66, 67, 71
Human Immunodeficiency
Virus (HIV) 47, 52, 63,
67, 76
Hyde, Byron 28, 32

IL-2 *see Interleukin-2*
immune system 18, 20, 21,
22, 26, 32, 41, 46, 47, 49,
51, 52, 53, 54, 55, 56, 57,
58, 59, 60, 61, 62, 65, 66,
67, 71, 72
influenza *see flu*
Interleukin-2 58
IQ drop 41, 71

Jessup, Carol 36

Klimas, Nancy 47, 50, 51, 52,
55, 58
Komaroff, Anthony M. 36
Koop, C. Everett 28, 29, 68
Kopanoff, Donald E. 75
Krueger, Gerhard 31

LEM 72, 73
lentinan 64, 72, 73
light sensitivity 38
Lloyd, Andrew 31
LNKS *see Low Natural Killer*
Syndrome
Lottenberg, Steven 41, 42
Low Natural Killer Syn-
drome (LNKS) 31, 72;
see also natural killer cells

ME *see myalgic encephalo-*
myelitis

Other Books By Neenyah Ostrom:

What Really Killed Gilda Radner?

Frontline Reports On The Chronic Fatigue Syndrome Epidemic

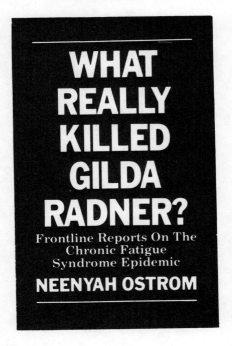

Available from:

TNM, Inc.
P.O. Box 1475
Church Street Station
New York, NY 10008

$14.95 (plus $3 shipping and handling)
400 pages   ISBN: 0-9624142-1-2